# ACHES AND PAINS SECRETS

## THE HIDDEN HEALTH CODE TO GET RID OF YOUR PAIN BY DE-STIFFENING JOINTS IN YOUR BACK

Chongsu Lee

# PRAISE FOR ACHES AND PAINS SECRETS

"The therapy devised by Chongsu improved my mobility, lifestyle and kept me working at the career I love. It changed my life. This book will change yours."

—Alison Peebles

Hardcover ISBN: 9798437601396

Paperback ISBN: 9798437588451

To my wife, Soo, for keeping me sane
through all my crazy work, for being
a wonderful mom to our son Geo and for standing by
me
as I pursue my dream of making the world a healthier
place.
To my dad, who always prayed for me
to be happy in whatever I do.
To my mom, who taught me not to agonize about the
things in life I can't change,
but showed me how to be a hard worker and earn
respect


In memory of Kerry Napuk (1939 - 2014), who showed
me the way

# CONTENTS

\* \* \*

Section 4

Secret Ten

Conclusion

# FOREWORD

## A MARRIAGE MADE IN HEAVEN...

I met Chongsu in 2015 at his treatment center in Edinburgh. I had read an article about his revolutionizing treatment for pain and mobility. I was in need of support and relief for both at the time in a big way. I had been diagnosed some years back with Multiple Sclerosis. I have always been up for trying something new, taking a chance and figuring out the best way forward no matter what circumstances you find yourself in. Chongsu Lee's treatment and background certainly fitted those criteria. I was intrigued by what I had read. An engineer turned physiotherapist from South Korea caused a tidal wave of interest and enthusiasm in Scotland with a unique treatment for pain and mobility issues. I wanted to find out more.

From our first meeting at his treatment room in Edinburgh, I was hooked. It was such a unique approach Chongsu used and he himself was different from any of the other therapists I had met. And in my quest for health and a decent quality of life I had met many! I was captivated by his background being engineering in South Korea yet here he was practicing physiotherapy in Edinburgh. His treatment of repetitive pushing movements along my spine became the focal point of my week. They were comforting, restorative and energizing treatments. But one a week was never enough and as much as I looked forward to the drive from Glasgow to Edinburgh it took its toll through the winter months.

It came as no surprise when Chongsu told me about his idea to build a robotic machine that could replicate the manual treatment. Ingenious was my first reaction. Only Chongsu Lee could come up with the idea to marry together the skills of his contrasting professional journey- engineering and physiotherapy- and invent a life-changing machine. One that you can have in your own living room. In your own bedroom. One that could influence and alter your life choices and quality. The idea may have sounded too good to be true to some. But they hadn't met Chongsu Lee. I had and I knew he could do it. I knew it would work and I knew it would change people's quality of life for the better. And it did.

This book takes you on Chongsu's compelling journey. He has been driven to help others for years and years. His invention of the BackHug is simply sublime. You have to experience it to believe it and then watch the positive impact it has on your mobility and pain discomfort.

I have become great friends with Chongsu over the years. We share a synergy to do things that can make life better. BackHug certainly does that and it has been my greatest privilege to be part of the whole project. I have benefited so much from the ingenuity, expertise and love that Chongsu spreads everywhere he goes. You can too now thanks to BackHug and this book. This book will uplift you. It will certainly motivate you and it will give you hope and belief in a better future for yourself. Just like Chongsu Lee himself, it delivers on its words.

—Patricia Gachagan

*Glasgow born Patricia Gachagan is an amazing, inspiring woman. It has been my privilege to know and to treat her. She was diagnosed with Multiple Sclerosis (MS) after giving birth to her son Embracing a new spiritual journey, Patricia continues to live her life with creativity, adventure and positivity. Her courage and determination are movingly expressed in her powerful memoir BORN TOGETHER (2017).*

# A NOTE TO THE READER

I started writing this book and came up with the original framework for my aches and pains secrets while my team and I were at the early stage of launching a tech startup. We were developing a therapy device designed to help people suffering from the aches and pains I write about in this book. After many years, the team eventually completed the development of a smart piece of hardware called BackHug (mybackhug.com). BackHug is my baby and this book explains the fundamental healthcare principles that are embodied in that baby, the journey I took to discover those principles, and how they can empower you to deal with your own severe aches and pains yourself.

Over the seven years that I served as a physiotherapist and as the founder and inventor of BackHug, my team and I could observe a really striking gap between the life changing improvements experienced by people who treated their pain with the "Joint De-Stiffening" methods outlined in this book and those who couldn't or wouldn't.

Most of the people I met, as a therapist and as a

quite a few were based on sound principles that helped me get even healthier. Those new insights encouraged me to do more research and actively manage my health. Having suffered so long as a child, I discovered that there was something I could do about it. So … I did something about it, and that set me on the path I have followed for the rest of my life.

# THE PERILS OF GOCHUJANG

It took me three years, but one evening after sharing pork ribs and kimchi with my friends Seol and Baek, I suddenly realized as I was going to bed - I don't feel sick. No acid.

When people ask me, "what cured you?" I can't offer them a silver bullet. What I can tell you is that it didn't happen overnight. Over time, my habits improved. I ate regular meals, cutting out spicy food as well as artificial ingredients, sugar and other unhealthy stuff. I continued the good habits I'd acquired at the start of my degree: Tai Chi, jogging, lots of meditation and mindfulness. And I tried not to worry (not easy, I know), to be more positive, appreciative and less sensitive.

I know none of this is particularly revolutionary and I'd be surprised if you hadn't come across some of these ideas before. The point is that it was those well known healthy habits that guided me to an understanding of what caused my problem in the first place. Having that rubber tube in my nose, taking drugs three times a day for almost ten years, missing school days, not being able to go out with my friends - I really hated it and I wanted to know why it happened.

Thinking back over those years, I understand the context a little better. My parents did what any parent who isn't a trained clinician would do - they took me to hospital. But what the hospital had to offer was no better than a band-aid. The acid the tube was pumping out was just a symptom. As that acid was pumped out, more just kept coming in again. I couldn't fix the root cause of the problem because no one knew what it was.

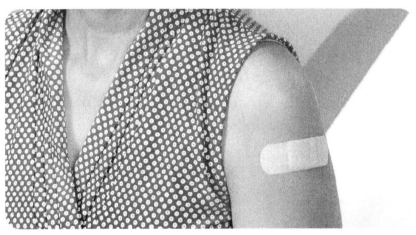

*Figure 0.1: The hospitals my parents took me to used a 'band-aid' treatment approach, which didn't address the root of my health issues.*

So…what was that root cause?

When I was nine, something terrible happened.

But not to me.

My brother Jongho was involved in a bad car accident.

My mother spent most of her time in hospital with him that year (thankfully he survived). I was left in the care of my father.

My parents were farmers and, as anyone who has worked on a farm knows, it's hard to look after a small boy when you're tending crops. So while my father was in the fields, I would go to the fridge and help myself to Gochujang, a red, ketchup-like saucy paste beloved by us Koreans. I craved Gochujang because it was sweet. That sweetness makes it kind of addictive - especially to a nine-year-old.

But it's also powerfully spicy, and it was that spice that damaged the lining of my young stomach and digestive organs.

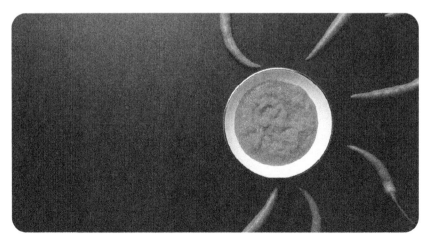

*Figure 0.2: When I was 9 years old, my mom was away for a*

*whole year and I ate lots of Gochujang - a sweet, spicy and addictively tasty sauce beloved by Koreans, which quickly damaged my fragile digestive system.*

So the acid that later needed to be pumped from my stomach was blowback from the time I spent as a kid living off Gochujang after my brother's car accident. Over the three years from when I started university to when my health finally improved, I spent a lot of time (and money) eliminating the things that were harming my digestion while adding anything that could help it. I was steadily turning the vicious circle into a virtuous one.

My take away from this process of experimentation and learning was that there's nothing worse than spending all of your time, energy, and money dealing with the symptoms of sickness or chronic pain without ever getting lasting relief by tackling the root cause. Is that something you can relate to?

We all want to live a happy and healthy life.

So when you spend every day fighting - just to not be in pain, just not to suffer, just to achieve a level of health most people take for granted - it becomes exhausting mentally, emotionally, physically, and financially...

Especially when your health never really improves

and you feel like you're just running to stand still.
That's when you can lose hope.

# TURNING POINT

But I was lucky. Somehow, I managed not to give up. Eventually, after years of effort, things slowly started to change. …

I liked Tai chi so much that it got me into other sports. For the first time in my life, I was getting fit. I also started researching what I was eating, learning more and more about what I was putting into my body and what effect it had. That was eye opening. I tried several different diets, including - at one stage - going for a month eating nothing but grapes (by now you may be thinking I'm nuts (pun intended), but the grape diet and the retreat on which I followed it were based on sound principles and did wonders for my digestion).

Month by month, I was eating more and more healthily and getting to know what was good (and not so good) for me.

The research I was doing into my diet was mostly trial and error. But that's how I discovered that the root cause of the acid in my stomach was a bad diet and lack of exercise. It took a while, but eventually I put two and two together to figure out that the Gochugang was the culprit for all that time I spent in hospital.

It was only once I knew what had caused the problem that I was able to focus on the solution. By changing my diet and exercising regularly, I was eventually able to tuck into that pork and kimchi - and really enjoy it - without paying the price afterwards.

# MY MISSION:
# FIXING THE ROOT CAUSE OF
# OUR HEALTH ISSUES

My experience didn't make me an expert in digestion.

But it did create a strong bond of empathy in me with anyone suffering because of their health. It also made me realize that a lot of healthcare is just a band-aid, like the tube in my nose. Too often, the healthcare we receive doesn't go to the root of the problem and leaves millions of people like me going back for the same drug, the same treatment, sometimes for their whole life, without ever getting better. If I was to pick out one thing that I gained from my suffering as a child and subsequent discovery of what caused that suffering, it's the determination to seek out the ROOT causes of any problem I encountered - especially health problems.

After graduation, I started my career as an international trouble-shooting engineer for Hyundai's automobile division in Seoul. It was intense. My experience was that the work involved spotting engineering problems before they got out of hand, as well as (more often than not) fixing them if that didn't happen. We always seemed to be scrambling to meet urgent deadlines - this is known at home as 'bbali bbali (hurry-hurry)' syndrome and is stereotypical of us Koreans (the "bb" in "bbali" is pronounced half way between a "b" and a "p") - anyone who comes to Seoul will quickly notice that everyone there is in a bbali bbali rush.

Although I loved the problem-solving side of engineering, my heart was somewhere else. So I found myself studying meridian massage in my spare time with Master Donhyun Lee, founder of the Korean Yakson Society ("Yakson" means "medicine hands" in Korean). As part of the program, along with fellow volunteers, I would visit care homes after work and on weekends to give Meridian massages to their elderly residents.

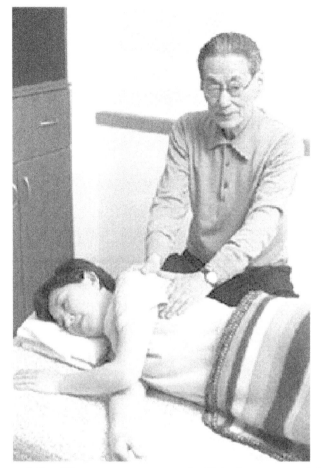

*Figure 0.3: Photo courtesy of Shindonga article on 29/01/2014. In my spare time, on top of my day job as an engineer, I spent time learning about meridian massage with Master Donghyun Lee*

That work as a voluntary meridian masseur planted the seed of my vocation. It was something I kept thinking about as I was working in Alabama and Georgia, helping launch Hyundai's first made-in-

America car. Two years later, I gave up engineering and took the plunge. I flew to Edinburgh, Scotland, where I had made some friends, to start again from scratch and study physiotherapy.

The technical knowledge underlying the information you read in this book is based on my years of clinical experience as a physiotherapist in Edinburgh. What led me to gain that experience was the Gochujang I ate when I was nine.

My experience as a sufferer and practitioner doesn't mean I have all the answers. But my illness and my physio training have taught me to recognize patterns in people suffering from a great many different kinds of pain and to use those patterns to identify the root cause of their suffering.

It has been my privilege and my joy to use this approach to help people regain their health and live their lives to the full. It is my mission to give hope to anyone else suffering from chronic health issues like I did.

I hope this story of my journey from a sick child to a physiotherapist who can heal people can inspire you with hope and positivity. Each case study in the book describes a unique problem faced by one of my patients and a unique insight that I gained while resolving that problem.

Each of those case studies relates to commonly experienced, typical problems which are likely to affect us at some point in our lives. Therefore, I recommend reading the whole book from beginning to end - you owe it to yourself to take a few minutes to end years of chronic pain. So get comfortable and take the time to read these secrets that I know will make a real difference to your health.

As you read through the case studies below, you will find a common thread to all of the problems I encountered in my patients and the solutions I found.

What underlies that common thread is a fundamental principle I discovered through my work. I believe that principle is the key to virtually all of the pain we experience in our muscles and other parts of the body like the head.

Although that principle is consistent with what you will find in textbooks, it hasn't been written down or articulated in any textbook. Until now, that principle only existed in the practice of individual physiotherapists and other healthcare practitioners. They did it, they knew it worked, some of them even authored manuals showing their specific techniques, but they never articulated the principle behind their practice.

By revealing the secrets in this book and the closely

guarded know-how that underlies them, I want to open the floodgates, so everyone has access to these life-changing insights and so anyone can experience a happy, empowered and pain-free life. I wrote this book to put that know-how down on paper and make the fundamental principles behind my secrets accessible to you. Knowledge can change your life.

The pain in your body is a call for help. We need to respond to it quickly, not ignore it. It's telling us to do something, to take action and change things, whether in terms of our physical or emotional behavior.

While most people try to run away from the pain in their body, or worse, to hide it with painkillers, wise people throughout history have seen pain as a sign. They listened to what that sign meant for them and figured out a way to solve it. Every improvement in your health starts in this way, I believe.

As the 13th-century Persian poet Rumi said:
"The cure for pain is in the pain."

This may be the most famous of Rumi's quotations, and it's a sentiment we can all relate to. Rumi's words hold truth. The cure for pain is often found within its depths, so don't give up … the treatment could be a simple tweak you haven't found yet but to which your pain can lead you.

I wanted to write this book because I know there are people like me who have been trying to restore their health and well-being yet are still struggling to live the healthy, pain-free life they deserve.

So many people I know try to alleviate their pain just by treating the symptoms and are frustrated when that doesn't get them anywhere. But there is a better way. It took me years to discover and master these secrets - but when I did, I was able to help people much more quickly, improving my success rate from 50% to almost 80-90%.

This book is the culmination of a decade spent experimenting and analyzing thousands of patients and their success stories. I have treated so many people suffering from an enormous range of problems and studied the methods of numerous therapists who successfully helped their patients day in and day out, by treating the root of the problem.

I hope that after reading this book you will realize that your goal of a pain-free life is a lot closer than you think. Soon, you'll discover that by recognizing the importance of getting to the root causes of your pain, understanding and applying the key principle behind my aches and pains secrets to that pain, making a few easy tweaks in your life, and committing just a little bit of time and effort, you can achieve a pain-free, healthy life. The ultimate goal of all of this is for you to get your life back, so you can spend your time and energy on the things that matter most to you and make you happy. By reading this book, I hope you reach that goal.

Before I start, one important note…

The names in these case studies have been changed to protect the anonymity of my patients.

Now, without further ado…I present the first of 10 life-changing secrets to help you discover the source of your pain and how to fix it.

# SECTION ONE

"Get the fundamentals down and the level of
everything you do will rise"

—Michael Jordan

## SECRET ONE
# THE ISSUE IS NEVER THE ISSUE

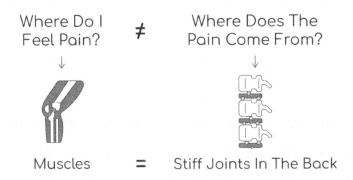

Where Do I Feel Pain? ≠ Where Does The Pain Come From?

Muscles = Stiff Joints In The Back

*Figure 1.1: First, you must ask yourself - Where does the pain come from? In most cases, the part of the body where you feel the pain is not the part where the problem causing the pain is located*

During my early work as a sports physiotherapist for Dunfermline Athletic Football Club, I looked after many junior players aged 10 to 19. One day, Alex, a shy brown-haired midfielder, came in complaining about a tight right hamstring. He struggled to stretch correctly, even though he spent 10 minutes on his routine before every game. The tightness in his hamstrings was making him slow on the pitch.

This was threatening his hopes of ever playing professionally. He was even scared that his hamstrings would snap one day, putting him out of the game for two months at least.

The first couple of times he visited, I went over how he was doing his stretching. From what I could see, he was doing all the right things.

When I checked him over, it didn't seem like anything significant was wrong with him.

So I did the obvious thing. I massaged his tight hamstrings using my thumbs and elbows, which gave him tangible relief.

Or so I thought…

… until he came back to the clinic for a third visit, and things were back to square one. This frustrated him and puzzled me. What was making this 17-year old's hamstrings so stubbornly tight? Another hamstring massage wasn't the answer. That would have been the equivalent of the tube in my nose for Alex.

"The definition of insanity is doing the same thing repeatedly and expecting a different result."

You've likely heard this quote, right?

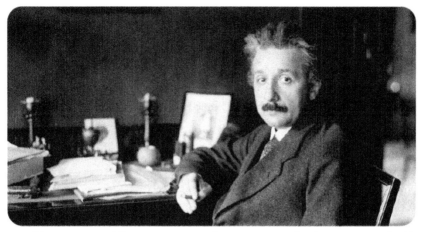

*Figure 1.2: Albert Einstein (1879 - 1955) physicist and all-round genius to whom many quotations are wrongly attributed.*

It wasn't going to fix his problem if I just kept doing the same thing.

I needed to think about the root cause of Alex's hamstring tightness from a broader perspective.

So I decided to check other parts of his body, including his back and his posture, to see if I was missing anything.

At the time, I was working crazy hours every day treating patients, and that intense manual work helped my hands develop an intuitive ability to quickly locate any joint stiffness or muscle tightness in a patient's body, kind of like a sixth sense. Using my hands, I assessed Alex's neck, back, legs and even buttocks to find any joint stiffness or muscle tightness.

Although it was very subtle and not obvious…

One crucial distinction caught my attention.

When I gently pressed my hands onto his lower back on the right, Alex responded with discomfort, even though his lower back was fine on the left.

Unsure about this potential connection between the slight twinge in the lower back and Alex's hamstrings, I repeated the test twice, which showed consistent discomfort in the right - but not the left - lower back.

So, instead of the usual hamstring exercises or muscle massage, I pressed my two thumbs onto his lower back joints to release their stiffness for 30 minutes.

I could tell he was getting confused.

"Why are you massaging my back, Chongsu?" Alex was not convinced about my treatment and was clearly starting to question my competence.

"It's my hamstrings that are sore, not my back…it's not like I'm going to score goals with my back, is it?"

 "That's a bit cheeky Alex. It's me doing all the work. You're just lying on the table." I said.

After half an hour of continuously applying pressure to Alex's lower back with my thumbs came the moment of truth.

I stopped treatment and asked Alex to get up and walk to see if he could feel any leg difference.

After just a few steps, Alex couldn't believe it

"My thighs - they're not tight anymore, Chongsu!"

He tried the hamstring stretch by bending forward. His fingertips went down by more than 10 cm compared to what he could do before the treatment.

The symptoms of tightness were in his thighs, but the root cause was in his lower back.

# WHAT DOES THE LITERATURE SAY?

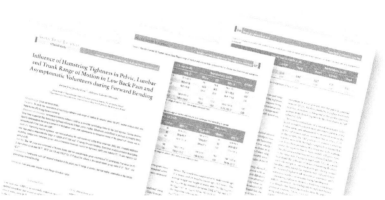

*Figure 1.3: Many studies show the relationship between tight hamstrings and lower back pain or hip pain*

While I was thrilled with these results, I felt conflicted.

This methodology was the opposite of what they taught me in college.

So, that night, I went online to see if there was any research on the relationship between lower back pain and tight hamstrings. To my surprise, there were enough studies to fill a bookshelf that demonstrated precisely that relationship.

There was just one problem.

Almost all of the literature I came across (e.g. Mistry and Vyas 2014, Reis and Macedo 2015) only went in one direction. They hypothesized that tight hamstrings caused lower back pain, not the other way around (as I had just experienced with Alex). Accordingly, they claimed that the solution for tight hamstrings was to stretch or massage … those tight hamstrings. Try as I might, I couldn't find any literature on that relationship that looked at the cause and effect the other way around. In other words, I couldn't find any researchers saying that a stiff lower back could cause tight hamstrings.

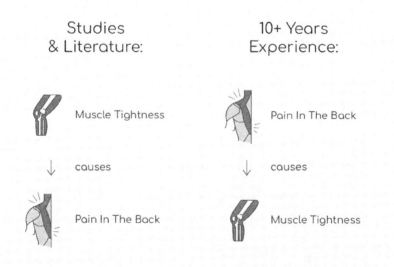

Studies & Literature:

Muscle Tightness

↓ causes

Pain In The Back

10+ Years Experience:

Pain In The Back

↓ causes

Muscle Tightness

*Figure 1.4: Most studies say tight muscles cause problems in the back, but in my 10+ years of manual physiotherapy experience, I found the opposite was true*

Alex is not alone.

The only treatment that is widely offered to people with tight or painful limbs is treating the parts of their body - almost invariably the muscles - around the problem limb. And, I must admit, that's pretty much what I did when I started practising as a physio.

But, as time went on, I became convinced that - except for direct injuries to the arms or legs or certain specific medical conditions (e.g. Stiff Person Syndrome or SPS) - most of the pain people experience comes from stiffness and tightness in their neck and back.

Are you surprised?

I was initially, but the more people I saw in the clinic, the clearer it became. The pain you experience in your neck and back can cause problems throughout your body, like Alex's hamstrings.

When left untreated for a while, which is what most of us tend to do - thinking the problem will just go away - pain which starts off as a minor niggle can easily become debilitating for your physical and mental health as time goes on.

This is a critical piece of knowledge if you want to naturally heal your body and get rid of your aches and pains. Without it, so many people waste so much time and money treating the muscles in their arms or legs, mistakenly assuming that's where their problem is, when the solution is to fix the joint stiffness in their back, which is the problem's root cause.

# TAKEAWAY SECRET

Instead of foam rolling, stretching or massaging your leg muscles, check with your therapist first to see if there is any joint stiffness in your back.

I guarantee you it will save you a lot of money and time.

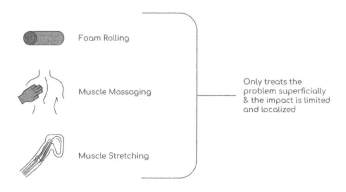

Foam Rolling

Muscle Massaging

Only treats the problem superficially & the impact is limited and localized

Muscle Stretching

*Figure 1.5: Foam rolling, massaging muscles, stretching muscles, massage chairs, and massage guns treat the problems superficially. At best, the benefits are short-lived*

Behind the solution to Alex's injury lies a broader insight: where you feel the pain is usually not where the source of the pain is to be found. I will develop this insight in the following chapters with specific examples.

My hope is that this insight will save you time. Instead of being distracted by treating the part of the body where you feel the pain, you'll be able to go straight to the source of that pain and find a lasting solution faster and more effectively.

So many people want to get rid of their pain, and they just start getting their muscles massaged, stretched or strengthened without really understanding the source of the pain. If you truly want to fix your pain, you need to start thinking differently and learn to understand it. Once you do that, you'll be able to identify where the problem comes from and figure out how to solve it quickly.

# TAKEAWAY EXERCISE

To start off, I want you to spend two minutes answering the following two questions.

**Where am I feeling my pain?**

If the answer is that you feel pain in more than one location in your body, then you can be confident that the source of that pain is in another part of your body. Or, if you are suffering from aches and pains in two or more locations of your body, and you feel as though those pains are related in some way, the source of the pain experienced in those different locations is probably in another part of your body and not in any of the multiple locations where you feel it.

**What did I try that worked and what did I try that didn't work?**

Be honest with yourself. Some of the things you tried may have felt good at the time. But how soon did your problem come back after you did that stretch, that exercise or that treatment? It doesn't matter how prestigious the profession or the therapist practicing that profession are, whether they are massage therapists, physical therapists, chiropractors, osteopaths or craniosacral therapists. It's really about where the therapist focused their treatment and how they treated the area. Remember all of those therapies, stretches and exercises are there to do a job for you. That job is to fix your problem so you can be healthy and pain-free. If they don't do that in a way that lasts, they're just another "band-aid." It's no better than the tube I had in my nose (see "Backstory" above). But if something really did work for you, if you felt sustainable improvement from any particular activity or therapy, think about which parts of your body were loosened. Not just the parts that were treated but other places in your body that also benefited. That may give you a clue to where the ultimate source of your pain is, which can help you not just target the stretches, exercises or therapies you go for but also make adjustments to your lifestyle, such as how you sit at your desk or lift your shopping.

I hope you now appreciate how important it is to understand that the source of your pain could be different from where you experience it. If you do, that's already a great start. Unfortunately, most people stop here and don't know how to take the next steps.

But if you want to find out what those next steps are, read on. The following secrets are designed to help you use your knowledge about the sometimes elusive source of your pain to identify that source and - crucially - treat its root causes.

## SECRET TWO
# ALL ROADS LEAD TO THE SPINE

Jane is in her 50s now.

When she came to see me, she had endured severe aches and pains and muscle soreness over the previous nine years. She looked tired, though she always tried to put on a smile. 'Work is stressful' she told me, 'not to mention bringing up three kids with no help from Alan.'

At first, the thing that stumped me with Jane was that her pain didn't seem to have any identifiable source. She hadn't experienced any specific injuries. Instead, it was as if her body had developed severe aches and pains like a rash in multiple parts of her body, making her tired and even more stressed.

Many people like Jane visit clinics every day, wondering where their pain comes from …

A lot of them don't have a diagnosed medical condition …

So they simply try to alleviate their symptoms with painkillers and we know how bad that is for you …

Many of them suffer in silence, never discussing how bad their pain is with anyone. Most of the time, these coping mechanisms do more harm than good.

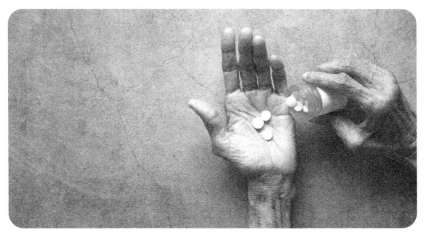

*Figure 2.1: If you don't address the root cause of the pain, simply taking painkillers usually does more harm than good*

Almost everyone experiences some form of pain at some point in their lives. For some of us, it's an occasional, possibly minor annoyance. For others, it's a chronic issue that requires medication (or so they think). Many people don't realize that simply taking painkillers without addressing the root cause of their pain can worsen the problem in the long run.

But things turned out differently for Jane.

They also turned out differently for me. My treatment of Alex (Secret #1) had already taught me to look beyond the part of the body where he felt the pain for the solution to that pain, but Jane's floating, shapeless pain was a new, even more critical, revelation. It took me directly to what I now believe is the source of most of the severe aches and pains we experience.

Jane had been coming to me (and other physios before me) for regular massages on the muscles in her back and legs for years. The relief that treatment gave her was welcome, but only lasted a day or two. After some soul searching , it finally struck me that maybe massaging her muscles might only be treating her symptoms, just like the tubing in my nose that sucked the acid out of my stomach. It was time for a different approach and I started to think about what might be the root cause of her pain.

But trying to find that root cause was like catching a blob of mercury. There was no pattern in the muscles where she reported feeling sore. There were no obvious clues for me to start my detective work.

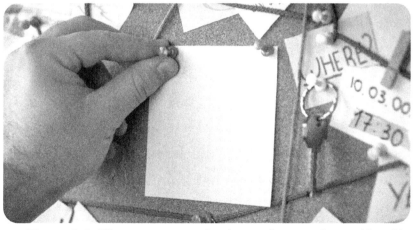

*Figure 2.2: The root cause of pain can be complex to identify, and it sometimes appears there's no apparent pattern to what*

*causes it to get better or worse*

Stiffness around joints in the back: But one dull day in April, when I gently pressed around the joints in her neck and shoulder blades, her reaction was different: she felt a distinctive discomfort that was much worse than what she felt in the muscles around the rest of her body. That told me that her neck and back joints were almost certainly stiff. It struck me that the joints there might be stiff, which might in turn be making the muscles surrounding those joints tight. Feeling tightness specifically in the joints is not always easy, you need a lot of experience. But when I checked the joints, sure enough, they were very, very tight.

# A MOST TEDIOUS TREATMENT TECHNIQUE

So I tried something simple. I gently pressed my thumbs around the joints in her neck, shoulder blades, upper back and lower back for thirty minutes, using a simple, repetitive motion which has now become my signature physiotherapy move. I don't know what made me do it. Perhaps I had spent so long looking for the problem that my brain was like scrambled eggs and couldn't think of anything more complicated. Maybe, under pressure, I was regressing to my engineer self, applying an almost mechanical, piston-like approach.

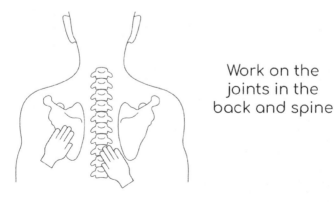

Work on the joints in the back and spine

*Figure 2.3: I worked on Jane's joints around her spine - neck, shoulder blades, upper back, and lower back. I applied pressure through my two thumbs to mobilize those joints and reduce their stiffness*

At the time, I wasn't optimistic. How could something so basic impact a problem so complex? I wouldn't have blamed Jane if she'd never come to see me again after such basic, repetitive, simplistic treatment for her lifelong muscle issues. While I pressed away, I could just imagine the conversation she would have with Alan when she came home.

Her: "You'll never believe what he did. He just pushed my back with his thumbs. The same thing, again and again."

Alan: "Uh huh."

Her "And again!"

Her "And again!!"

Alan: "Uh, that's it?"

Her: "Pretty much."

But the results were surprising for both of us (and Alan, I assume). After the session, the unfocused shards of pain that Jane had felt throughout her body had dissipated.

Could this be luck?

Placebo?

Nothing else had worked, so I decided to continue with the same approach.

(I know what I said about the definition of insanity and doing the same thing expecting a different result, but this was different. I was doing something that had worked and hoping for the same result, which I'm sure Einstein would have approved of).

Also, I was a little curious...

What if this monotonous, primitive approach was the key to something bigger?

What if I had cracked a massive secret to pain relief that doctors and specialists had missed?

After a few sessions, to my amazement, the experiment kept replicating the same result.

Jane's symptoms kept improving, just from repeated, mechanical mobilization around her spine.

Before I get carried away, readers should bear in mind that the pain many people suffer from is the result of a complex combination of factors, often involving a history of injuries or emotional trauma. This is what often makes treating pain so difficult: even if you address one issue successfully, there may be other factors that need serious attention and of which you have no knowledge. What if Jane was experiencing a great deal of stress at her work or in her marriage? That could easily have negated the beneficial effects from my treatment. In Jane's case however, I was lucky: she was managing the other factors that might have contributed to her pain very effectively, and that made my therapy work really well for her.

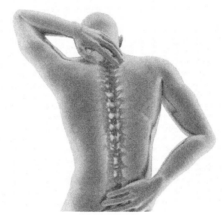

*Figure 2.4: The spine, lying in the center of the back, is a "highway" connecting the head, face, arms, chest, stomach, neck, hip, legs and foot to each other. The spine holds many little-known secrets to our health.*

It's hard for me to describe the profound sense of fulfillment I get from helping people like Jane, who have been suffering for years, trying everything but still living in pain, day in, day out (maybe that's because I'm an engineer: I'm used to communicating in diagrams and bill of materials spreadsheets, not emotions).

But having spent most of my childhood in pain due to my digestive issues, I knew how they felt. You never get used to chronic pain. It takes over your life and becomes part of the fabric of your everyday existence. You can't imagine a life without it. So the overriding feeling you have is one of hopelessness.

What made me tremendously excited about the results I got with Jane was that I had stumbled upon an approach that might give hope to people like her, after years of living in pain with no prospect of any solution.

There are three simple ways of moving and loosening your joints:

Exercise and stretching

Manual treatment (like the one a skilled therapist would perform on patients like Jane)

Treatment on a magical device that replicates the manual treatment I used on Jane (that magical device was in development at the time, but I'll come back to it at the end of this book).

## How To Lubricate Stiff Joints

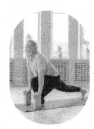 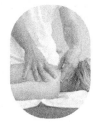 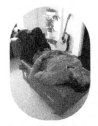

Exercise
& Stretching

Manual
Treatment

Treatment Using
a Device

*Figure 2.5: Three different ways you can lubricate the stiff joints in your back*

# WHY DOES LOOSENING JOINTS WORK SO WELL?

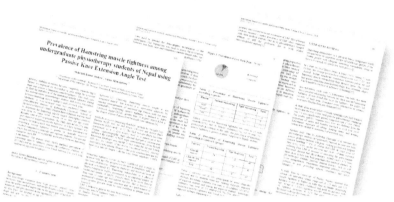

*Figure 2.6: Many studies identify a relationship between muscle tightness in the back and different kinds of pain. But it's hard to find any studies explaining why relieving stiff joints can alleviate those forms of chronic pain*

The stakes were high. Although Jane's experience was encouraging beyond my and her expectations, she was only one patient. Could this approach work more widely? To answer that, I had to dig deeper into the theory. Finally, I had found something that worked - the "what?"

Now I wanted to start understanding the "why?"

Specifically…

Why can something as simple as treating the joints in the back result in such a life-changing outcome?

I read the literature, looking for an answer to that question. The first thing I encountered, which had always struck me as odd when I was doing my physio training, was how little scientific literature there is on the subject. Although lower back pain is the single largest cause of global disability according to the World Health Organization[2], very few clinical studies investigate the more specific relationship between, say, joint stiffness in the back and chronic pain in the leg.

This is for several reasons I think. First, people can't measure pain or discomfort. It's pretty subjective. They can't give me an objective figure or measurement of pain because everyone experiences it in different ways at different times.

Moreover, many factors might contribute to your pain - lousy posture, wearing a bag on your shoulder or picking your kids up every day - whose impact can't be measured precisely. And back pain is so familiar and ordinary that it may not excite researchers in the way studying the effects of a molecule on a rare form of cancer might.

When I studied the literature, I (re)discovered that

_____

[2] World Health Organisation, Musculoskeletal Health (July 2022), https://www.who.int/news-room/fact-sheets/detail/musculoskeletal-conditions

pain in the back is understood to be closely related to muscle tightness in the hips and legs. According to numerous studies (Shakya and Manandhar 2018, Hasebe et al. 2016), issues in the muscles - in the buttock or hamstrings for example - can severely affect the hips and lower back joints. Moreover, those studies showed that treating tightness in the muscles will relieve pain around the joints (see Tak et al. 2013).

But, just as when I re-opened the textbooks to understand what was happening with Alex, I couldn't find any studies exploring whether the relationship might work the other way around.

This seemed really strange to me.

When I was working on Alex I had seen that treating muscle tightness in his legs did nothing or very little for his back.

How could it, I remember thinking? That causality didn't make sense.

But treating the stiff joints in his back had transformed the tightness in his legs.

You don't need to be Dr Sajin Tak to understand that if the joints are stiff, they will exert pressure and pull on the surrounding soft tissues and neighboring muscles, through which vital nerves travel, making them tight.

When I say it like that, it seems like common sense,

doesn't it?

As my career progressed and I started to build a network among my fellow practitioners, I came across a handful of other therapists who had noticed the same relationship and embedded it in their practice. So I'm not claiming to be the only person who has discovered this, and it's reassuring to know that what I'm saying is supported by other experienced practitioners. But here's the thing. I think that this principle is too important to be contained in the isolated know-how of a few scattered practitioners. It deserves to be more widely known. It should be accessible to you - and to everyone.

# A SECRET HISTORY OF JOINTS

To understand why my treatment worked, I'm going to have to talk about joints, which is not a topic that people think about much. Muscles are much easier to relate to, we think of "muscling in on something," "flexing muscles," "muscle memory," "I want muscle" by Diana Ross ... The same with "bones" - "I feel it in my bones," "show some backbone," "you're all skin and bones," "a bone-crunching tackle," "Daddy Cool" by Boney M ... ok, sorry, no more dad jokes in the rest of this book, I promise. But joints kind of get overlooked. Is there any common phrase we associate with joints? I couldn't think of one. They just sit there quietly, connecting our bones to each other, not attracting attention to themselves.

What I discovered while I was researching the topic, for my practice and for this book, is that joints are just as overlooked in scientific literature as they are in our common phraseology.

So here is the secret story of why stiff joints are the

root cause of most of the pain we experience. To tell that story, I'm going to lay out five key therapy concepts, which, combined, answer that question. After that I'm going to explain how loosening those stiff joints can help with your pain as well as your health in general.

# KEY CONCEPT #1:
## ALL MECHANICAL PAIN IS A RESPONSE TO STRETCHING OF, OR PRESSURE ON, THE NERVES

To understand why the joints are so important for pain, you need to understand what causes pain in the first place.

The gold standard physiotherapy textbook by F. P. Kendall and his colleagues, in its 5th edition at time of writing, Muscle testing and function with posture and pain (Kendall et al. 2005) clearly states that 'whether it is in the muscle, the joint, or the nerve itself, pain is a response of the nerve. The mechanical factors that give rise to pain must directly affect the nerve fibers.'

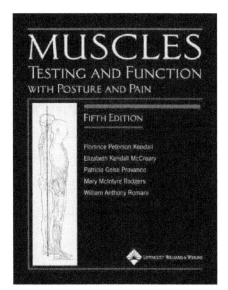

MUSCLES

TESTING AND FUNCTION
WITH POSTURE AND PAIN

FIFTH EDITION

Florence Peterson Kendall
Elizabeth Kendall McCreary
Patricia Geise Provance
Mary McIntyre Rodgers
William Anthony Romani

LIPPINCOTT WILLIAMS & WILKINS

### MECHANICAL CAUSES OF PAIN

Pain—whether it is in the muscle, the joint, or the nerve itself—is a response of the nerve. Regardless of where the stimulus may arise, the sensation of pain is conducted by nerve fibers. The mechanical factors that give rise to pain must, therefore, directly affect the nerve fibers. Two such factors need to be considered in problems of faulty body mechanics.

Pressure on nerve root, trunk, nerve branches, or nerve endings may be caused by some adjacent, firm structure, such as bone, cartilage, fascia, scar tissue, or taut muscle. Pain resulting from an enlarged ligamentum flavum or a protruded disk exemplifies nerve root pressure. The scalenus anticus syndrome in cases of arm pain and the piriformis syndrome in cases of sciatica are examples of peripheral nerve irritation.

Tension on structures containing nerve endings that are sensitive to deformation, as found in stretch or strain of muscles, tendons, or ligaments, can cause slight or excruciating pain, depending on the severity of the strain. Forces within the body that exert an injurious tension resulting in strain of soft tissue usually arise from a prolonged distortion of bony alignment or from a sudden muscle pull.

*Figure 2.7: Kendall' book is a physiotherapy bible and there it states 'whether it is in the muscle, the joint, or the nerve itself, pain is a response of the nerve' But, few therapists practice on this basis*

Mechanical pain means pain caused by significant stress or strain on the muscles and/or joints, typically caused by things like bad posture, sitting too long, awkward lifting or bending motions. It is distinct from pain due to illnesses (e.g. cancer pain) or blows (like cutting your finger with a knife or hitting it with a hammer). Both Kendall and my experience as a physio agree: almost all of the chronic mechanical pain we experience is the direct consequence of pressure or tension on the nerve.

In addition to this insight, at physiotherapy college,

I learned a concept called 'neural tension.' The term describes what happens when nerves are not sliding and gliding through tissues as they usually would. Instead, nerves get stretched because there is pressure or tension on them. This neural tension is what puts pressure on the nerves and it is pressure on the nerves, as Kendall says, that causes mechanical pain. It's a concept that fits with what I have observed as a practitioner.

This way of understanding what causes pain, based on the concept of 'neural tension,' is backed up by evidence, although, interestingly, the evidence for treatments which try to reduce neural tension is mixed (Walsh, 2005). I'm pretty sure that's because the most common physiotherapy treatments for 'neural tension' symptoms are stretching exercises that try to help the affected nerves glide through the congested soft tissues, such as median nerve gliding exercises for Carpal Tunnel Syndrome (Ballestero-Pérez et al., 2017). But after reading my case studies you shouldn't be surprised to find out that those standard treatments are not that effective.That's because the neural gliding exercises don't address the root of the problem, which is joint stiffness in the back. To be fair, it's really hard to treat stiff joints in the back using a therapist's two thumbs (I discovered this to my cost, as I will discuss in later chapters), so I don't blame them for going for the easier soft tissue massage techniques.

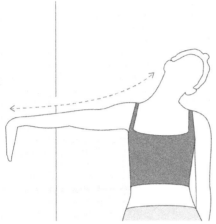

*Figure 2.8: Median nerve stretching is a standard physiotherapy treatment for Carpal Tunnel Syndrome, but its effects are no better than the use of a wrist splint. This unimpressive outcome is due to the fact that the treatment doesn't address the root of the problem*

Simply put, the neural gliding exercises are another form of stretching exercise based on the "treat-where-you-feel" approach. In other words, they don't pay much attention to where the problem started in the first place - where the tension on the nerves is coming from. That's why so many studies find that nerve gliding stretches often have outcomes that are no better than basic injury management techniques, like using a wrist splint (L. Brininger et al., 2007).

But whatever you do to treat neural tension, one thing is clear: pressure on and stretching of nerves is key to all the mechanical pain we experience. Therefore, to fix your pain, you need to remove the pressure from those nerves.

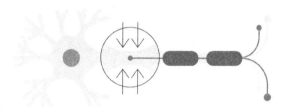

*Figure 2.9: Most of the pain we experience is a response to pressure on our nerves. So, to fix your pain, you need to remove the pressure from those nerves.*

Once we grasp this concept, the next question is 'where does that pressure on the nerves come from?' That's where the joints come in.

# KEY CONCEPT # 2:
# MOST PAIN IS CONNECTED TO
# THE JOINTS IN THE BACK

We also know that the spine is a superhighway for nerves. Indeed, the central nervous system (CNS) runs through the spine and connects the brain to the spine. The peripheral nervous system (PNS) which "includes all of the 31 pairs of nerves that branch out from the CNS, i.e. brain and spinal cord" (Soames et al. 2006) extends to the rest of our body, including shoulders, arms, hands, hips, legs and feet. In other words, all nerves either run through the spine (CNS) or are connected to nerves that run through the spine (PNS).

CNS                    PNS

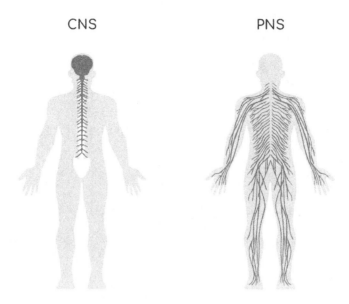

*Figure 2.10: All nerves either run from the brain through the spine (CNS) or are connected to the CNS. And all nerves connected to the CNS go from the spine to the arms, legs, chest and everywhere else in the body (PNS)*

But before all those nerves in the PNS leave the spine to travel to the rest of the body, they have to pass through a gate. That gate is the spinal joints in the back. In reverse, when nerve signals from the arms, legs, neck and even the back itself enter the spine, they have to pass through the joints in the back. No surprise then that most of the pain we feel as a result of nerves being stretched or stressed are connected to the joints in the spine.

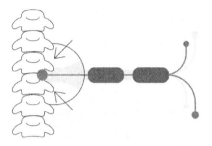

*Figure 2.11: The stress on your nerves almost always comes from the joints in your back. That's because the nerves in your neck, back, arms, and legs all start from the joints in your back*

# KEY CONCEPT #3:
# THE JOINTS IN THE BACK ACT AS SHOCK ABSORBERS WHEN THE BODY UNDERGOES STRESS

The next question is 'why does pressure congregate in the joints in our back?' Although, in theory, the obstruction can happen anywhere along the course of the nerve, human anatomy and biomechanics clearly indicate that almost all pressure or tension on nerves involves the spinal joints in the back.

First, let's look at how our body is constructed to understand why the joints in the back suffer the most.

Here is an important statistic. Our neck and back have more than 150 joints! Just to put that number into perspective, there are only two joints in the knee, two in the ankle, and four in the shoulder and around 200 in the whole body outside the back. In other words, the back has about as many joints as the rest of the body combined.

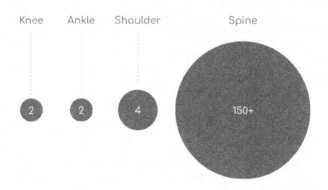

*Figure 2.12: Our back has around as many joints as other parts of the body. Each joint in the back can become stiff, and the impact can travel across the whole body.*

Each of those 150+ joints in the back can become stiff, and if multiple joints that are close to each other become rigid at the same time, that can make your back and neck a disaster zone, littered with stiff joints, one on top of the other.

Interestingly, when our ankle gets stiff we notice it pretty fast and usually don't wait too long before visiting a therapist.

That's only for two joints.

So just imagine the impact on our body when about 150 joints in the back become stiff.

But we don't notice the tension in the joints in the back as much as in the ankle, even though there's over 50 times as much of it. That's because it's - literally - at the 'back,' behind us, where we can't see it. It's also because our back is much less sensitive than other parts of our body, like our head or limbs.

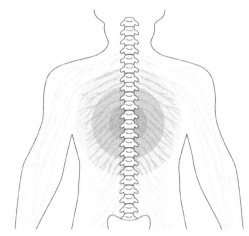

*Figure 2.13: The back is anatomically right in the middle in the body, and is designed to support the movement of the head, arms and legs*

Furthermore, the back is where our spine, or "backbone" is, and it acts as the backbone of our whole body structure. You can bend, turn, and rotate your head because your head is sitting on top of your back, connected by your neck. Similarly, you can type on a keyboard using your arms, or kick a ball with your legs, because both your arms and your legs are held securely onto the back (via the pelvis in the case of the legs). In other words, we can move our head, arms and legs in all sorts of fluid and flexible ways thanks to the fact that our back is there in the middle, sturdy and stable, holding everything together.

The back is designed to provide stability to the body so that the head, arms and legs can do what they need to do. As a result, when our body experiences physical stress, it's our sturdy and stable back, and our spine, that absorb that stress. Whether you are sitting for 8 hours working away at a computer desk or driving four hours in your car, your back always takes the most strain. Every human being on earth feels the weight of gravity and it is our backs that hold us upright under that weight.

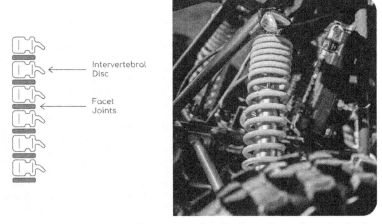

*Figure 2.14: Joints in the back are shock absorbers for the body. When physical strain is experienced anywhere in the body, the shock almost always goes through the 'shock absorber' joints in the back, travels through the spine, and leaves the spine through*

*the 'shock absorber' joints in the back again*

In turn, it is specifically the joints in the back that cope with the stress that is soaked up by the back (as described above). Joints are flexible, so they can absorb the force and stress experienced in the back, reducing the negative impact of physical strain on the other bones in the back (Ocran E., 2022). Bottom line: the joints in the back are like a reservoir, into which flows most of the stress our body experiences.

# KEY CONCEPT #4:
## STIFF JOINTS IN THE BACK CAUSE PAIN NOT JUST IN THE BACK BUT IN OTHER PARTS OF THE BODY

That's not all.

The joints in the back are all connected. They're like a water pipe. If any part of that pipe becomes blocked, it will block the whole pipe. Similarly, stiffness in one part of your back, whether it's in the neck, shoulder blades or upper, middle or lower back, will affect the entire back. That means working on one or two joints is usually not enough, because even the most experienced therapist can completely miss the particular joint in the back that really matters - and the "pipe" will still be blocked. Also, if they're lucky enough to find the right joint, they would need to spend at least 20 minutes to treat just that one joint to have a meaningful impact on it.

* * *

And that's still not all. Stiff joints in the back don't just cause problems in the back. The stress absorbed by stiff joints in the center of the back are only the beginning. Their impact travels through the whole body.

To explain how this happens, I need to introduce you to a little known part of our anatomy and investigate mechanisms in our bodies which haven't attracted much attention from researchers up to now. Physiologically speaking, problems spread from our back to the rest of the body because our entire body is connected through a type of connective tissue called 'fascia'. Fascia connects everything in our body together; (Adstrum et al. 2017 and Dalley et al. 2006). Facia are a type of connective tissue in our body that behave like a long roll of double sided tape, extending through our body to hold or "stick" everything inside it together: bones, muscles, nerves, blood vessels, ligaments, tendons, organs, and everything else. Without fascia, our body would fall apart, just like the Nebula character in Avengers: End Game.

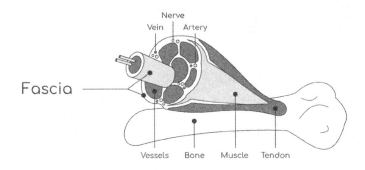

Nerve
Vein | Artery

Fascia

Vessels   Bone   Muscle   Tendon

*Figure 2.15: Fascia holds everything inside our body together: bones, muscles, blood vessels, nerves, and everything else. Fascia is incredibly important but little studied.*

You can think of the fascia in our body as a large sheet of tablecloth. If you pull it at one corner, that pull will affect the entire tablecloth, although the extent of the impact will obviously vary depending on how hard and the distance from where you pull. It is very encouraging to see that a growing number of medical doctors and healthcare institutes are beginning to recognize the importance of fascia and integrate them into how they treat their patients (Brennan, 2021). A couple of health textbooks, both published in 2014, focus their advice on the health of the fascia: Move Your DNA by Katy Bowman and Born to Walk by James Earls.

The joints are supposed to be loose and "well

oiled" with Synovial fluid - a thick liquid located between the joints - to allow movement. But, if they get stiff as a result of stress as described above, it makes the surrounding connective tissues, the fascia, tight. In turn, those tight fascia apply pressure to the muscles and nerves. This means that injuries or tightness in one part of the body can easily cause issues in other parts of the body. As the tension in fascia ripples through other parts of the body, the 2nd, 3rd, and 4th nerves become stretched through the tensed fascia and develop pain.

# KEY CONCEPT #5:
## STIFFNESS INTERRUPTS THE FLUID FLOW OF NERVES AND BLOOD VESSELS

Even though fascia are crucial, they're not the only means of transmission of that stiffness.

When stiff joints in the back make the surrounding muscles tight, as described above, the nerves and blood vessels coming out of those joints get squeezed by tight soft tissues and muscles. As a result, the nerve transmission and blood circulation to the head, shoulders, arms, and legs both become compromised.

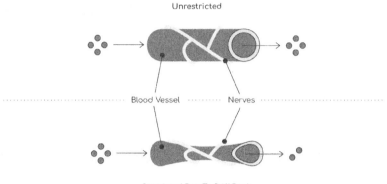

*Figure 2.17: Joint stiffness in the back causes muscle tightness, which in turn interrupts the fluid flow of nerve transmission and blood circulation.*

You can easily experiment quickly with what happens when your body's nerves and blood vessels struggle to flow freely. Hold your wrist with your hand and squeeze it firmly. I tested this on my friend Christopher. He was one of my physio patients and soon became a good friend, along with his friend Kerry (we'll come back to Chris and Kerry in Secret #10, in which Kerry played a key role). To illustrate the concept, I squeezed Christopher's right wrist with my hand.

"Can you make a fist?" I asked.

"I can do that … but my fingers feel stiff" said Christopher.

"I'm going to squeeze it even more firmly. Now, try

again please."

"My fingers feel much stiffer now, it's hard to move them properly." Christopher acknowledged.

"What else do you feel?" I asked

"It feels kind of tingly and it's starting to hurt. In fact it's becoming really painful now. Chongsu … can you please let go?" As soon as I released my grip, the pain rapidly subsided and he could move his fingers normally again.

What was happening when I was squeezing Christopher's wrist was that the nerves and blood vessels there were tightening. That's what made it hard to move his fingers and caused the pain and tingling sensation.

Although it was Christopher's wrist I was squeezing, the same principle applies to the back. By choking off the transmission of the vital sensory information conveyed by the nerves and the circulation that runs through the blood vessels, stiff joints in the back can cause all sorts of problems all over the body: headaches, hamstring tightness, tennis elbow, Achilles tendonitis … I could go on for pages and pages. This underlines the central point (pun intended) - starting from the center of your back, the consequences can be felt all over your body, transmitted by the nerves and blood vessels.

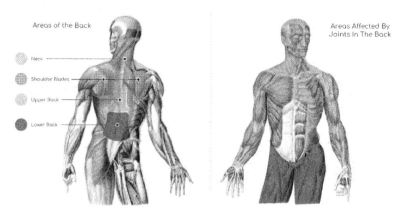

*Figure 2.18: Our back is divided into the neck, upper back, shoulder blades and lower back. Each of those areas affects different parts of the rest of the body*

Our back is divided into four main areas:

1.  Neck
2.  Shoulder Blades
3.  Upper Back
4.  Lower Back.

Each of those areas affects different parts of the rest of the body.

For example, the problem in Alex's legs was caused by the stiffness in his lower back. This explains why injuries, aches and pains in so many seemingly unrelated parts of the body can be traced back to - and be fixed by treating - the stiff joints in the back.

# SUMMARY:
# THE DOMINO EFFECT

The way the pain travels in our body is like a domino effect. Joint stiffness in the back causes discomfort in the affected joint area first. Then, it creates tension in the surrounding soft tissues, including fascia and muscles. The tension, through the ripple effect in the fascia, nerves and blood vessels travels to other parts of the body. As a result, the pain spreads across the neck, shoulders, upper back and lower back, travelling as far as the head, arms and legs (as we saw with Alex). This is different from what happens if other parts of your body, such as your ankle or elbow, get stiff. In those cases, the problem only affects the ankle or the elbow and doesn't travel to bother any other part of your body.

This is important because if you want to fix the pain in your arms and legs, or your headache, or even your tennis elbow or Achilles heel, you need to go to where the problem started in the first place - that is, almost invariably, the stiff joints in your back!.

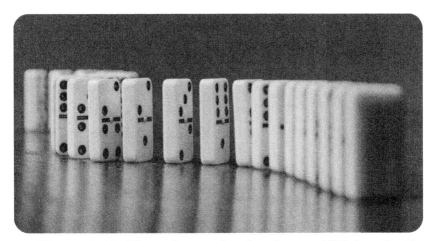

*Figure 2.19: The aches and pains from stiff joints in the back are only the beginning. They travel through the whole body in a domino effect.*

Putting all key concepts #1 to #5 together and the following conclusion is unavoidable:

When our body experiences stress and physical strain, the joints in the back take most of the stress because the back is where that stress and strain are absorbed and the joints are the back's 'shock-absorbers' (Key concept #3)

Stiffness in the joints in the spine will make the surrounding connective tissues, the "fasciae," tight and taut, which applies pressure to the nerves around the spine. (Key concept #4)

Spinal joints in the center of the back are also the

nexus for all peripheral nerves (PNS). (Key concept #2)

The nerves coming out of the spine are densely connected to the rest of the nerves in the body and any pressure or tension they experience will be transmitted throughout the whole body. (Key concept #5)

Neural tension theory explains that pressure or strain on the nerves will cause pain on those nerves and all the nerves that branch out from them. (Key concept #1)

And all mechanical pain, according to Kendall, is "a response of the nerve." (Key concept #1)

Therefore, nearly all mechanical pain has its origins in stiff joints in the back.

I want to underline this once more as it's a crucial point. The gold standard of physiotherapy principles agrees with me that all mechanical pain, whether it is in the muscle, joint, or ligament, is solely caused by compression and stretching of the nerves elsewhere in the body, not by factors in the muscle itself.

Furthermore, according to the basic biomechanical principles of neural tension, stiff joints are a key reason why nerves become stretched and compressed in the first place.

From there, it's a short step to put those fundamental insights together. Combining those insights, we get a robust validation for the key principle in this book: most mechanical pain is caused by joint stiffness in the back and shoulder blades where the nerves start their journey.

## Fact 1
From Kendal, et al

___

All mechanical pain is caused by pressure or tension on nerves.

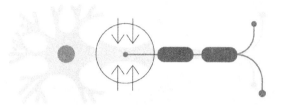

## Fact 2
Based on "Neural Tension"

___

Almost all pressure or tension on nerves starts at, or involves, stiff joints in the back.

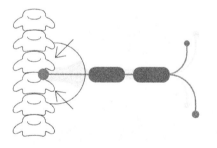

---

### Our Secret:
Almost all mechanical pain is caused by stiff joints in the back

---

*Figure 2.20: If we put the insights together - (1) the insight about pain being caused by pressure on the nerve (from Kendall et al.'s book and neural tension theory) combined with (2) the insight that the spine is where all the nerves go to and also where most of the joints in the body are placed - we get a robust conclusion: all mechanical pain is caused by, or involves, stiff joints in the back*

# STIFF JOINTS ARE LIKE
# A RUSTY BICYCLE CHAIN

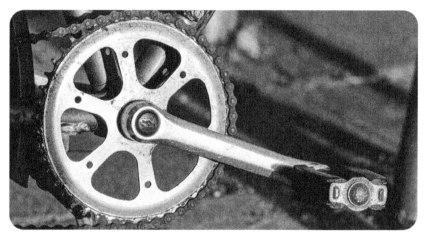

*Figure 2.21: Just as a bicycle chain can become rusty, our joints become stiff, which makes them hard to move. The rusty bicycle chain needs oil and so too do our stiff joints need us to restore their natural movements.*

You may be wondering, if stiff joints are the problem, why is loosening them the solution?

The analogy I find helpful is to think of the joints in our back as being like a bicycle chain. Your bicycle chain gets rusty when you leave it out in the rain for too long. If the chain is rusty, it doesn't matter how good the wheels are or how hard you pedal, the bike will grind along slowly, making an unpleasant noise.

Similarly, the conclusion I came to was that the joints in our back become "rusty" because we:

- Get older, especially after 40
- Sit too long at a desk
- Get stressed
- Pick up injuries or suffer falls

.

After treating hundreds of patients, I went on to believe that the impact of stiff joints in the back will expand throughout the rest of the body.

When the joints in the back become stiff, we need to "pedal harder" to move our body. Joints even make noises from time to time, a characteristic clicking sound. So, it dawned on me that, just as you would put oil on a rusty bicycle chain to get it moving smoothly again, you need to "lubricate" your joints if they become stiff - to get your body moving smoothly again.

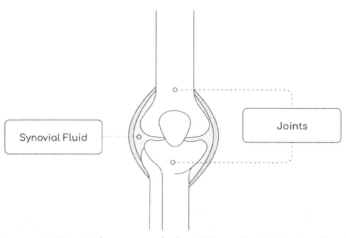

*Figure 2.22: When we feel stiff and tight in the back, physiologically, it means that the amount of 'Synovial' fluid in the joints may not be sufficient, making the joints a bit 'dry' and, causing joint stiffness*

The best way to "lubricate" stiff joints is to move them gently. But how do we know that?

Due to the limitation of existing measurement technologies, such as Ultrasound and MRI, most people accept that scientists have so far struggled to prove that the volume of joint fluid, or, to be precise, 'Synovial' fluid (described above in Key Point #4) increases as a result of joint mobilization work (Trijffel et al. 2016). However, most experienced physiotherapy teachers - those who train future physiotherapists in college - teach on the assumption that joint mobilization helps lubricate the joints in the back. And it kind of makes sense, intuitively, that moving joints should loosen them. This is one of many areas in which common sense and the know-how and practical experience gained by working in the field have reached a conclusion with which the science will eventually catch up when measurement technologies improve.

What hundreds of thousands of physiotherapists have worked out from over a century of practice is that by moving joints, you ease the pressure and tension in the surrounding muscles, as well as in the ligaments, tendons, nerves, and blood vessels. As a result, the Synovial fluid fills the space around the joints and literally (yes, literally!) lubricates them, allowing them to move smoothly again. The benefits of the lubrication we achieve in the joints by moving and loosening them in this way then spread throughout the body.

# HEALING MODE VS. FIGHTING MODE

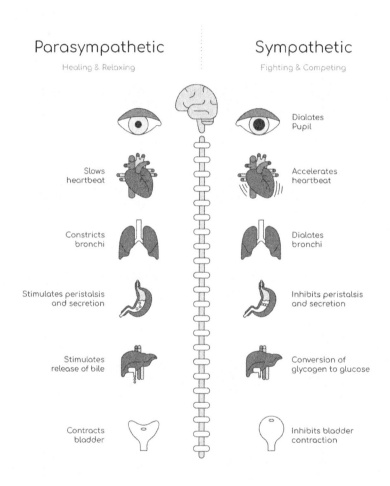

*Figure 2.23: Sympathetic nervous activity enables us to fight and compete. Parasympathetic nervous activity restores, rests, heals and lets us sleep and smile. Any effective treatment must promote Parasympathetic nervous activity*

\* \* \*

The key to why my treatment works for physical pain is, as we saw, intimately connected to the nerves. I have also become convinced that the impact of my treatment on the nerves affected more than just my patient's experience of physical pain. In other words, there's more to it than joint lubrication.

In particular, the nerves that run up and down the spine carry out two types of activities, one termed 'Sympathetic' and the other 'Parasympathetic.' Those are perhaps odd names to describe what our nerves are doing, so let me explain.

In simple terms, Sympathetic nervous activity is what our bodies use to activate our "fight or flight" response.

It's useful for competition, work and crisis management. It comes into its own on the sports field or if you're a competitor in The Apprentice or Shark Tank, for example.

Confusingly, Sympathetic nervous activity is on the opposite side of the spectrum from the part of our personality we use when we're expressing our "sympathy" for others.

Contrary to Sympathetic nervous activity, Parasympathetic nervous activity enables us to be peaceful and relaxed. It stimulates our body to produce hormones that help us cool down after all the arousal of the Sympathetic nervous system.

Parasympathetic nervous activity gives us our "me time," it enables the R&R which is critical for healing - whether from illness, injuries, pain or even grief. One of the reasons massage feels good and is good for us is that it stimulates Parasympathetic nervous activity.

Crucially, Parasympathetic activity is shown to increase when we treat the stiff joints in the back (Kingston et al., 2014). Indeed, that happens whenever we get a back massage. I strongly believe that the therapeutic benefits of Parasympathetic activity are significantly increased when it is stimulated by any treatment that undoes joint stiffness in the back.

Now that we've seen how important the joints in the back can be, let's follow them to find the other - often surprising - parts of the body that may be causing you pain and discomfort.

# TAKEAWAY SECRET

Got a mystery problem causing you pain that you just can't solve? Go to the physio and get them to examine your back, asking them if they can notice any particular areas of stiffness. That area of stiffness in your back is almost certainly the clue you need to fix your mystery problem.

# SECTION TWO

"Life is really simple, but we insist on making it complicated"

—Confucius

# DON'T HANG YOUR HEAD LIKE A SNOWBALL

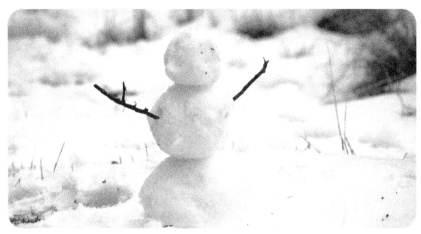

*Figure 3.1: The top snowball can fall off if it's placed off the center of the larger snowball below it. Even though your neck won't exactly fall off if it's off-center for a long time, it will put a lot of strain on your neck and shoulders)*

When I was growing up in Korea, we had lots of snow in winter. So, like most kids, I would go out with my friends to make snowmen and throw snowballs at each other (and, on one occasion, my elder sister's boyfriend, but that's another story).

I enjoyed stacking a smaller snowball on top of a larger one, imagining the smaller one as a head sitting on the larger one's shoulders. Maybe I was already playing at being a physio, who knows? It was fun, but it didn't amount to much.

The snowballs were uneven, and the small one never sat straight in the middle of the big one. So, it never took long before it started wobbling, sagged to one side, and eventually fell off.

Of course, it didn't matter because these were just snowballs. They would melt anyway (or get thrown at the boyfriend). But something very similar happens to our necks every day, and that matters a lot.

Our head is like a small snowball sitting on top of a bigger one. Unfortunately, like the small snowball, our heads can spend a lot of time sitting off-center. This may be happening to you right now if you're leaning forward to read this book on your computer or smartphone. Luckily, your head won't fall off when you do that.

However, the neck's joints, muscles and other soft tissues have to work hard to keep your head attached while you're leaning forward.

The longer you spend with your head in the off-center, "small snowball" position, the longer your neck's joints, muscles and soft tissue have to work. This makes the muscles tight and the joints stiff and misaligned.

An adult head weighs about 12 lbs on average. However, if you move your head even a little bit forward from where it is when you're keeping it perfectly straight, the weight bearing down on your neck increases dramatically. For example, when your head bends by as little as 15°, if you are bending forward to look at the menu on the table in a restaurant for example, the weight on your neck more than doubles, to 27 lbs (if you have an average weight head).

When the head bends by 30°, the impact trebles and the load your head is putting on your neck increases to 40 lbs (again, for an average weight head). In extreme cases, where the head is bent by 60°, the load on your neck increases to five times the weight of your head!

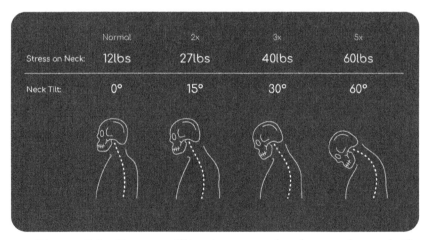

*Figure 3.2: Every millimeter your head goes beyond the central line, which represents good posture, the load on your neck increases dramatically. As a result, all the joints and muscles in your neck are forced to work much harder, and eventually get stiff and misaligned*

\* \* \*

As a result, the neck joints get stiff and go out of alignment.

No surprise, right?

The muscles get tight. The nerves and blood vessels around the neck joints become squeezed.

That is critical, because those nerves and blood vessels travel all over the body, to the head, face, shoulders, arms, elbows, wrists, and hands.

The neck is like the most significant highway interchange for nerves and blood vessels in the body. That's because the neck connects the head to the rest of the body. If that critical highway is blocked or damaged, it can cause significant pain and discomfort in your head and face (see Ogoke, 2000).

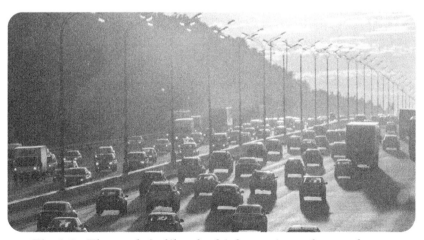

*Fig 3.3: The neck is like the highway interchange for nerves and blood vessels, connecting the head to the rest of the body. If that highway interchange is even partly blocked, it congests the*

*nerve transmission and blood circulations towards the head and face, causing headaches, brain fog and many other symptoms.*

If you're reading this chapter, there's a good chance you may have a stiff neck. So I hope you're sitting straight. You may have had it for a few months, or maybe for so long you've forgotten you had it. If that's the case, it wouldn't surprise me if you suffered from:

- Tension headaches (The most common type of headache, Hvedstrup et al. 2020)
- Pain in the back of your eye
- Brain Fog
- Feeling unusually tired, even after sleeping eight hours at night
- Compromised hearing (Zeigelboim et al. 2016)
- Even pain in your elbows or hands can be stiff neck-related.

# THE TOP OF THE NECK MATTERS THE MOST

In summer 2021, physiotherapist Aranzazu Lopez opened her physiotherapy clinic, coincidentally in the same building as the workshop in which I was developing a therapy device designed to replicate my manual treatment technique.

My colleagues and I were a bit puzzled at the time, because the Covid-19 pandemic that swept across the world since early 2020 was still front page news. Sure, more than 70% of the adult population was vaccinated, but a lot of people were still recovering from the scare and wary of close contact with other human beings for fear of infection. We thought her clinic might struggle to attract enough customers.

We needn't have worried. Aranzazu is a brilliant clinician. She knows what she's doing and within two months it was hard to get an appointment.

In fact, so many people had developed niggling pains and injuries during the pandemic - quite a few of them had probably been working from home at their kitchen table - that they were desperate for treatment.

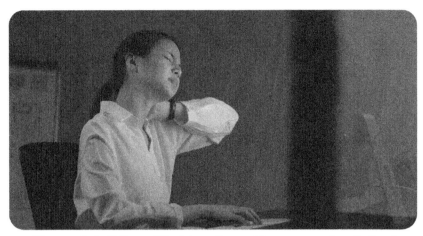

*Figure 3.4: When Working From Home, people sit for long hours, often in sub-optimal conditions, and are less active. As a result, many people started feeling sore or picked up injuries during the COVID19 pandemic.*

.

The 'Working From Home' or #WFH new normal made most people spend more time sitting at a computer desk. As a result, they became less active. They didn't need to walk to work or catch the bus. There were no colleagues to go to the gym with. As a result, many people developed poor posture.

Their neck and back got stiff. Their muscles became weak. Any sudden activity or exercise after spending so long in such a sedentary lifestyle will easily cause injury.

Aranzazu and I got to know each other well soon after she moved in, we're both outgoing and curious, and I invited her to try a prototype of the therapy device we were developing at the time. She had a few suggestions about how the product could get even better if we changed certain features.

Aranzazu moved from Spain to the UK several years ago and was passionate about her profession. I was impressed with her clinical knowledge and extensive manual therapy experience.

Aranzazu has spent 10 years training in three different, well-established fields of professional therapy: four years in physiotherapy, five years in osteopathy, and one year in chiropractic.

(Impressive, right?)

You can tell how enthusiastic she was as a clinician. Her customers couldn't praise her enough.

Of course, that made me all the more curious to know what she thought …

One day, I had a bit of a headache and wanted to check things out with Aranzazu to see what she made of it. I was also curious about how she would treat it. So, I booked in for a session with her.

"I feel a bit stiff in my neck and recently had some headache," I said.

"You of all people should know better," she scolded, "you've probably been working too much on the computer."

"I know… I know. I don't think it's anything serious." I replied, a little chastened.

After she checked a few things with my neck and head posture, she said

"The top joint in your neck is completely - well - jammed … I mean on the left."

"Oh really?" I didn't expect that. I hadn't felt the stiffness. "That explains the headaches I guess."

"That's it Chongsu. The joint at the top of your neck. It gets jammed really easily because your head is on top, no? So everything is not flowing right, you see, everything is, you know, blocked. So you are getting a headache."

She then worked on my neck joints to relieve the traffic jam, and after I stepped out of her treatment room my headache was gone.

If you're asking, do physios get treatment from other physios then I can let you into another secret on top of the ten in this book. Yes! Sure, we know all the exercises we can do ourselves (some of which I'm sharing with you in this book). But sometimes things are too tight, you're in too much pain and you just need a massage! When you're a physio, people sometimes assume you must be fit and healthy, and that you would never have any back pain. That assumption makes some physios afraid of talking about their own back pain and they often end up suffering in silence - I'm speaking for myself, and I'm sure it applies to many of my physio colleagues too!

Unfortunately, you can't massage the back of your own neck, it doesn't work - you just can't relax with your arms in that position and you would be constantly straining your neck and shoulders to perform the massage. We're basically like hairdressers - they can't cut their own hair, so they have to ask their colleagues (or even competitors). Similarly, when we need a massage, we have to turn to other physios.

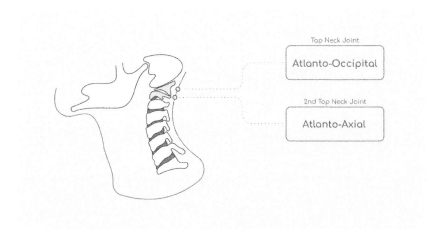

*Figure 3.5: The two top joints in the neck are the most important when it comes to treating a stiff neck. They become easily jammed, as they are right underneath the weight of your head.*

Not all joints in the neck are equally affected by

stiffness and misalignment.

For example, the top joints in the neck, which are just underneath the head, are most affected by prolonged sitting or smartphone 'texting' neck. When those top neck joints are jammed, people can experience all sorts of symptoms, including nausea, blurry vision, insomnia and even tinnitus (Ogoke, 2000). So, the most effective treatment for the neck aims at releasing that stiffness and fixing the misalignment in those joints.

# TAKEAWAY SECRET

If your neck is suffering from stiffness, it's likely because it's been sagging like a small snowball on a giant snowball. Although painkillers for headaches may seem like a quick fix, what you really need to do is relax the tension in the joints in your neck, especially the top of your neck.

Here's what you can do for yourself to self-release the stiffness and fix the joint misalignment in the top joints of your neck. If you suffer from a stiff neck, follow the exercise below daily, and your neck will feel looser and liberated (the exercise is from Dr Alan Mandell, see Mandell, 2016).

## Head Gliding

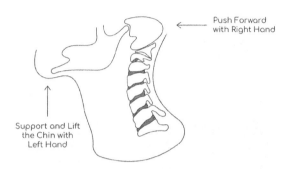

Push Forward
with Right Hand

Support and Lift
the Chin with
Left Hand

1. Support your chin with your left hand, place your right hand at the back of your head

2. Gently lift your chin with your left hand, while the right hand pushes the head forward, creating a gliding forward motion of the head. Repeat 10 times

3. Turn the head to the left, repeat 10 times

4. Turn the head to the right, repeat 10 times

*Figure 3.6: The "head gliding" exercise can effectively release stiff neck joints and restore misaligned joints, relieving many severe aches and pains experienced in the head and face.*

# HOW I SAVED MY MARRIAGE BY TREATING SCOLIOSIS

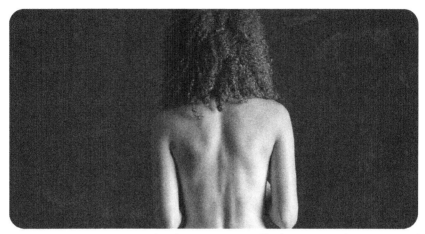

*Figure 4.1: Upper back sits vertically between the neck and lower back, as well as horizontally between the two shoulder blades*

My wife Soo used to complain that her shoulders were sore. And they were, pretty much every day. She also had headaches at least a few times a week.

Now I know what you're thinking.

She's married to a physio, what's going on?

You're probably feeling I must be a failure as a physio, as a husband, or possibly even both.

The embarrassing truth is that, by the time I got home from work most evenings, I was completely burned out.

After seeing so many patients every day…there was no gas left in the tank.

Especially as, most of the time, I was performing

the repetitive, mechanical work I used to help patients like Jane.

Try making the same pressing motion with your thumbs again and again with a short break between patients for an eight-hour day. You'll be lucky if you can mix your significant other a cocktail without dropping it.

Many of you - both women and men - will be able to relate to the struggle to make marriage and job both work. It's not easy. But in my case there was the added provocation that I was entirely qualified to help Soo; the only reason I couldn't (or wouldn't) was that I'd used up my energy helping other people.

It was bound to end badly.

One day Soo had enough. "For God's sake, do something about my shoulders and my headache!" Well, ok, that's not really what she said, but I want this book to be family reading.

So I slowly lifted myself off the chair and examined her back, shoulders and neck, just like I had been doing all day before coming home. After almost two years together, I'm embarrassed to say that this was the first time that I noticed that Soo's upper back was slightly curved to the left. The technical word for that curve is "scoliosis."

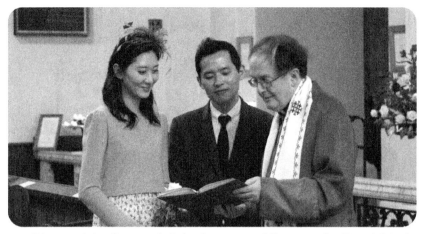

*Figure 4.2: Soo and I had our wedding at St Patrick's in Edinburgh*

When I touched the curved part, she screamed at me even louder than before.

The thing is, I love Soo. Being married to her is one of the greatest joys of my life. So, you can imagine how I felt, knowing that I'd missed such a blatant problem and had left her suffering.

And before you judge me too severely, I need to tell you something. From time to time, I would actually massage Soo's shoulders. I focused on her shoulders because that's where she felt sore. You're probably thinking that contradicts everything I've just been saying about the problem not being where you feel the pain. Guilty as charged, when I got home I would go back to the conventional way of thinking which I'd learned to avoid when I was practicing in the clinic.

Unsurprisingly, it never seemed to make much of a lasting impact. But seeing the curve made me think the way I did in the clinic. Was the soreness in her shoulders due to that scoliosis in her back?

I gently applied thumb pressure to her upper back joints to find out about the level of stiffness around her scoliosis - just as I would have done if she were a patient at my clinic. But the upper back is the most challenging part to work on (I'll explain how I do it and why it's so hard later in the chapter). I didn't have a treatment table at home for her to lie down, which made it even harder to properly treat her. But I had to do my best for Soo.

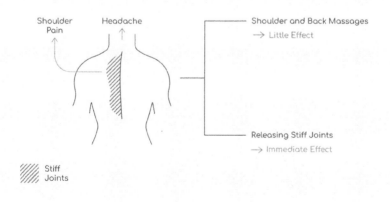

*Figure 4.3: When I massaged Soo's shoulders, it didn't do anything, but whenever I worked on her curved upper back, her headache disappeared*

* * *

Luckily, it worked so well that after just 20 minutes of treatment, her headache and shoulder pain went away. After that, I kept giving her the same treatment a few times a week, after coming home from work, and her shoulders stopped being sore. And she didn't leave me, so the hard work was worth it.

Knowing that the treatment wasn't just working in the short term, but that it was going to the root of the problem to produce a lasting benefit, gave me a sense of purpose that helped me find the energy to do yet another treatment after a long day at work.

Ideally, Soo would have benefited more if I were to have given her daily treatment, but I wasn't always available. We thought some of the massage tools heavily advertised on social media and television might do the job for her. So, Soo tried a massage gun, massage chair and massage bed, and quite a few other fancy massage tools in the bargain, but unfortunately none of them gave her any lasting relief. We ended up reselling them on eBay.

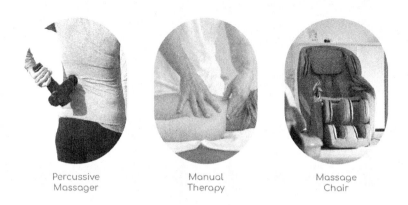

Percussive
Massager

Manual
Therapy

Massage
Chair

*Figure 4.4: Soo tried many kinds of conventional massage equipment available on the market to relieve her headache and shoulder pain, but none of them seemed to have long-lasting benefits*

As luck would have it, I later developed a device that did the work for Soo instead of me (this is the therapy device I alluded to when discussing my treatment of Jane and which I'll come back to in the last chapter). Soo started using my new device regularly by herself, and, within a few months, most of her aches and pains went away. She still uses it regularly to ensure the pain doesn't come back.

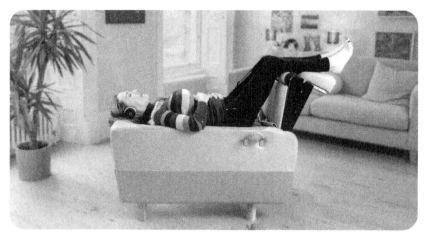

*Figure 4.5: Since using my new invention, Soo no longer suffers from aches and pains in her head and shoulders.*

# SECRET TAKEAWAYS

- If you have sore shoulders or headaches, there's a good chance that a stiff upper back is responsible for your problems.
- Remember, your shoulder muscles may feel tight, but massaging the tight shoulder muscles is unlikely to produce any long-term benefits to solve the shoulder pain (or headache).
- However, releasing joint stiffness in the upper back will really help keep shoulder pain and headaches at bay.

# THE MYSTERY STABBING CHEST PAIN

My friend Eric is in his fifties.

Unlike most men his age, he boxes. It's not that he's in denial about how old he is, but he's drawn to extreme forms of exercise that will keep him as young in body as possible for as long as possible.

One day when we were talking on a video call, he wasn't his usual self.

Something was obviously bothering him…

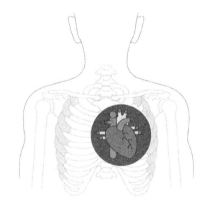

*Figure 4.6: Pain in the ribs may appear as if you have a problem in your heart*

He was subdued and didn't have his usual banter. I

could sense something was wrong. After a while he said that he'd suddenly experienced a stabbing pain between two of his ribs while he was at boxing training. Although it wasn't as intense as at the start, it was pretty sore and restricted his freedom of movement.

He had no idea where it came from

"Chongsu, there's no muscle between the ribs, you don't use that part of your

body for anything. How can it get sore like that?"

And worst of all, it was stopping him from boxing.

"Fitness for guys my age is like rolling a big boulder up a hill. You work hard for

months, even years, to get into shape. But if you get injured, you let go of

the boulder, and it rolls back to the bottom in a few seconds. A few weeks of missing training sets you back months in terms of fitness."

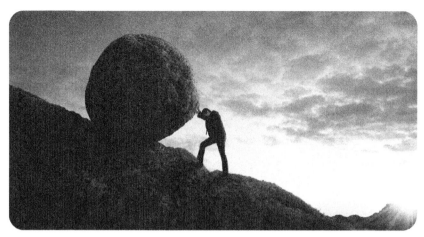

*Figure 4.7: When you are over 40, you need regular exercise to maintain your health, just like pushing a boulder upwards. Otherwise, your body may lose its health quickly, just like a boulder rolling back down the hill.*

Eric seemed to be less concerned about his actual pain than about not being able to train and losing his shape.

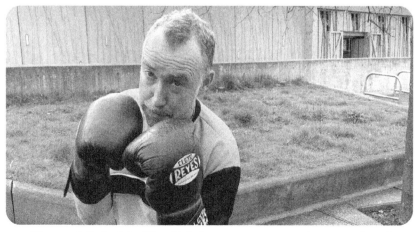

*Figure 4.8: In his 50s, Eric boxes once or twice a week to keep*

*fit. I recently joined his boxing training group - it's hard work!*

I sympathized with him. Not being able to do what you enjoy is depressing.

And while there are many different causes of pain, one thing is for sure: when your body is hurting, no matter where it hurts, it casts a cloud over everything you do.

Whether you love to swim, run, or box like Eric, pain can prevent you from doing the things you love.

I couldn't check his problems physically, so I advised Eric to give it a few weeks of rest as he may have hurt some of the muscles in his chest (contrary to Eric's belief that there are no muscles between the ribs, there are in fact many muscles around the ribs, albeit small "involuntary" muscles you can't actively control) during the intense boxing training. So, he did that.

Three weeks later, we spoke again and - the problem was still there. "Why does something so stupid take so long to heal! Waiting for this pain to go is like watching paint dry."

Eric had used acupuncture for various injuries over the years and enjoyed a good relationship with his acupuncturist Dr Ming, a formidable woman who had joined the Red Army at thirteen before coming to the

UK. In her 80s, she loves her job and continues to treat patients with unstoppable energy.

Eric is convinced she'll still be practicing fifteen years from now. She also has a soft, cat-like deftness when she plants her needles, and Eric hoped that if she planted a few in that stubbornly painful space between his ribs, he might be boxing again soon.

But Dr Ming took one look and said, with her characteristic bluntness, "your back is tight here and here," prodding Eric's upper back with her thumb.

"Your rib pain is from your upper back."

"Fact is," Eric later admitted, "I was being lazy." As a friend of mine, Eric is an early adopter of the new therapy device I invented and has an early version of it at home. But when it reduced the tension he had built up in his back from many decades of sitting at a desk (like many people in their fifties), he stopped using it.

Slowly but surely, the tension had returned and sat there, like a time bomb.

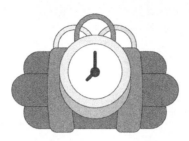

*Figure 4.9: Stiffness and tension in our back needs continuous management to prevent the development of severe aches and pains. If you don't do anything, the build-up of tension resumes, like a time bomb waiting to explode.*

It was only a matter of time until doing extreme exercise like boxing with a stiff back resulted in injury, and that injury came in the form of a sore intercostal muscle.

Since then, Eric realized that releasing the stiffness in his back requires regular work. He's not getting any younger, much as he tries, so stopping this "maintenance work" will encourage the problem to return on a regular basis. In addition, the "bicycle chain" needs ongoing lubrication from time to time.

Otherwise, it will get rusty again.

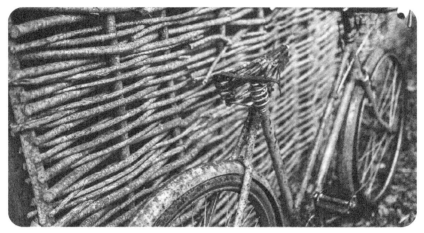

*Figure 4.10: The bicycle chain needs ongoing lubrication. Otherwise, it gets rusty.*

When your body, or parts of your body, feel fine, you can easily think that you can get away with not looking after it or them. But just because it isn't causing you pain doesn't mean it's fine.

The older you get, the more true the saying "prevention is better than cure" becomes. So it's important to stay active and maintain a regular stretching routine for your body, particularly your back. That will make you much less likely to pick up painful, long-lasting and annoying injuries like Eric's intercostal strain, which can set your fitness back a long, long way.

Now let's look at this mystery intercostal strain in more detail. Eric had a valid question. How could this bit of flesh between the ribs become so painful?

The clue is in the upper back. The upper back sits right behind your rib cage. And the rib cage is rigid. It has to be, to protect our heart and lungs. But that rigidity also makes the upper back hard to stretch off or to treat.

What does this have to do with the stabbing pain in Eric's chest? The answer is connected to the nerves and blood vessels that come out of the upper back and travel to the chest and shoulders.

When the upper back joints become stiff, the surrounding soft tissues and muscles in the back become tight. As a result, the nerves and blood vessels that travel through those tight muscles become constrained.

Some of those nerves and blood vessels reach all the way to the front of the chest, including the Pectoralis and Intercostal muscles. Disruption of the flow through those nerves and blood vessels can cause pain, numbness, pins and needles (as we saw in Secret #2). The stabbing pain Eric was experiencing in that bit of flesh between his ribs was caused by the impact of a stiff upper back on the nerves and blood vessels flowing into his chest.

Aches in your chest like intercostal strain can feel as though there was something wrong with your lungs or even your heart, which is a severe medical condition. But, in all likelihood, they are probably caused by tightness in your upper back.

In addition to stabbing pain in the chest and sore shoulders, signs that your upper back is stiff include:
- Stooped posture
- Chest twinges
- Shallow breathing (as opposed to deep abdominal breathing)
- Headaches

Luckily, some competent physiotherapists and chiropractors understand the critical relationship between a stiff upper back and various symptoms in the chest.

Since they see this connection, their treatment is focused on relieving upper back stiffness through manual therapy, exercise, or self-help methods. (LOR physical therapy, 2019.)

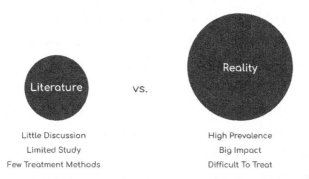

*Figure 4.11: There's hardly any literature acknowledging the importance of managing upper back tightness even though it's one of the most common physical presentations for almost everyone over 40, and its negative impact on our health is huge*

Unfortunately, there is hardly any literature on the impact of upper back stiffness. The most highly cited studies to mention the problem typically regard upper back tightness as a minor problem, which doesn't have a widespread impact (e.g. Eidelson et al. 2021). This attitude is reflected in the WHO's widely followed Global Burden of Disease bulletin, which is the ultimate source for our statement that lower back pain is the single largest cause of global disability (above, in Secret #2). It has data on low back pain and neck pain, but not upper back pain. For their part, most studies offer generic remedies like standard exercises or painkillers for issues such as intercostal pain. This leaves many people like Eric scratching their heads.

My years of manual physiotherapy experience helping all of my patients made me think differently, and I have a diametrically opposite conclusion to consensus. I think we have to accept that most people over 40 will develop a stiff upper back, often severely stiff, unless they do something about it.

It's also my experience that most of them don't know that their stiff upper back is the root cause of many of their most persistent health issues.

Unfortunately, my experience is that it was often only when a specific problem or injury flares up, and they're in severe pain, that my patients would seek help. The good news is that by treating the stiffness in their upper back, I was able to get surprisingly powerful results.

# TAKEAWAY EXERCISE

Now we know why having a stiff upper back can have such a wide variety of negative impacts, I want to show you how you can identify how stiff your upper back is. I have used this method to quickly assess my patients in the clinic. You can use that method for yourself by following the steps below.

If you're going to do this test, why not spend time with your family or friends and discover who has the stiffest upper back? Although experts tend to neglect the importance of upper back stiffness, I'm sure you'll all be surprised by how common it is.

## How High Can Your Thumb Reach When You Bring Your Right Hand Behind Your Back?

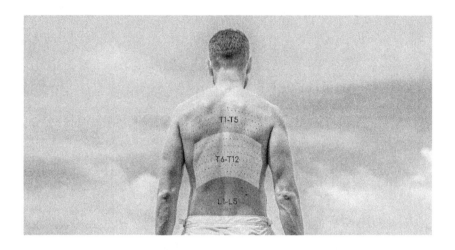

Zone 1 between T1 - T5
Zone 2 between T7 - T12
Zone 3 between L1 - L5

Repeat the same test with your left hand If two hands fall into either Zone 2 or Zone 3, you have a stiff upper back and may experience the symptoms described above

*Figure 4.12: There's a simple way of assessing the stiffness level in your upper back. The higher up your thumb reaches, the less stiff your upper back is*

If you discover that you have a stiff upper back, then it's time to release it.

I'll show you two ways to do that yourself.

* * *

Correct stooped posture: Just like the joints in the neck become stiff when the head and neck are bent and out of alignment (see Secret #3), stooped posture exerts harmful stress on the joints in the upper back. As a result, the upper back joints become stiff. So, the first thing you need to do is correct your stooped posture and try to stop any bad habits that contribute to the development of stooped posture.

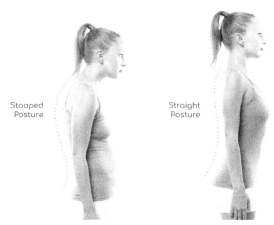

*Figure 4.13: The first thing you need to do to fix a stiff upper back is try to adopt good posture when you sit, walk or stand*

While there are many posture correction exercises you can do, I recommend trying a posture correction strap. You can buy them online. When you wear it at work or even when you're out walking, the straps prevent you from hunching forward and helps maintain an upright posture. They're not expensive, and it's a small investment that can pay off handsomely in a short period of time.

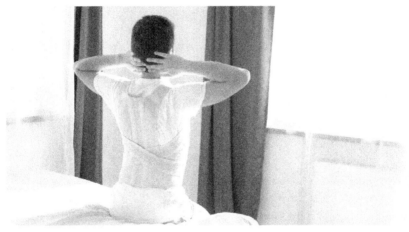

*Figure 4.14: A posture correction strap is a great way of preventing stooped posture*

De-stiffening the joints in the upper back: Get a lacrosse, golf or any small hard ball. Place one of the balls on the floor, and lay your back on the ball. Adjust your position so that the ball presses where you feel achy and tender near the spine in the upper back. Stay with the ball in the same spot until you feel the stiffness reduce and you can feel relief. Don't move the ball too quickly around your back. The benefits will be reduced if you do this. Only move to the next location where you feel stiffness once the first stiff spot has relaxed.

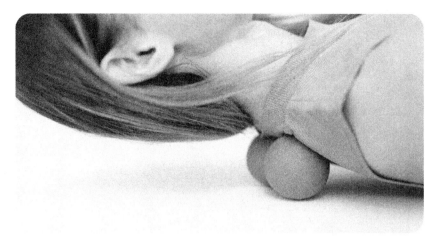

*Figure 4.15: Place a lacrosse ball underneath your upper back and rest on it. Stay still on it rather than bouncing about. If you stay for 1 - 2 minutes in one spot, you will feel the tension reduce, then you can move on to the next spot where you feel tight*

# THE STIFF SHOULDER BLADE TV TRICK

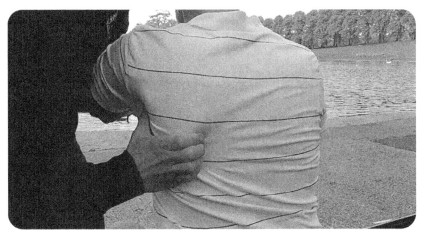

*Figure 5.1: In this blade treatment I grab the left shoulder blade from behind using my right hand, and then slowly move it to the right and left. This requires quite a bit of skill from the therapist.*

If you're like most people, you probably take your shoulder blades for granted.

You use them every day without even thinking about them.

But what happens when one or both of your shoulder blades becomes stiff?

One day while I was writing this book, I watched a health program on YouTube that I had first seen on television and had stuck in my memory. It featured Mr. Kim, who was introduced on the program as a "World Class Yoga Master," showing the audience, which included many health experts, how he could treat severe shoulder pain in one minute.

A female in her 40s was one of the first to volunteer. 'It's so bad I struggle to push my shopping cart. Even chopping potatoes is getting hard.'

The audience became emotional as she described how she fought through the pain because she was chopping the potatoes while making a meal for her kids. Mr. Kim proceeded to ask her to raise her left arm. When she did, she couldn't get her arm above shoulder level. That showed just how stiff her shoulder was.

Firstly, Mr. Kim performed a few tests on the movements of her arm and shoulder. Then he poked around her shoulder, upper back, and shoulder blade, her reaction clearly showing him that she was sensitive and sore there.

After a minute of checking, Mr. Kim said "The shoulder blade got stuck at the back. That's why you have shoulder pain."

He went to tell the audience that "the vast majority of shoulder pain is due to stiff joints in the shoulder blades."

Then Mr. Kim showed off his magic trick. He grabbed her shoulder blade from behind with his right hand. By moving her arm with his left hand, he went on to rotate the shoulder blade gently from left to right, then right to left,

The woman smiled momentarily before letting out a glass-shattering scream …

Mr. Kim's treatment was causing her a lot of pain. But about 30 seconds into the treatment, things started to improve.

Her face looked more comfortable, only frowning from time to time as Mr. Kim moved her arm from side to side. Finally, after a minute, time was up. Mr. Kim then asked her to raise her arm again.

To most of the audience's amazement and mine, her arm rose to her ear, twice as high as what she had managed only a minute ago. Everyone was impressed. Mr. Kim was just smiling.

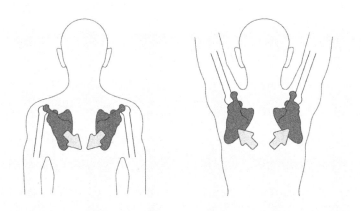

*Figure 5.2: The two shoulder blades are 'floating' over the rigid rig cage in the upper back. Any shoulder movement involves the rotation of shoulder blades, either inwards or*

*outwards.*

We have two shoulder blades, one on each side of the back. The shoulder blades are called 'floating joints.' That's because they are not like most joints.

Most joints are connected to other bones via multiple ligaments. But the shoulder blades are not connected to other bones. Instead, they "float" on the top of the rib cage. They are only connected to the rest of the body by a pool of muscles. That's why we say the shoulder blades are "floating" in the upper back.

Now here's the problem. The upper back's structure is rigid because of the rib cage (as described earlier). That means the shoulder blades have to slide over the rib cage when they move, from left to right. Because the upper back becomes stiff quickly (see Secret #4), that stiffness will impede the motion of the shoulder blades over time and make them stiff too.

What's more, stiffness in the shoulder blades impacts the rest of the body, just like stiffness in the upper back does. That's because the shoulder blades take up about 25% of the back area and so have many nerves and blood vessels running underneath them which travel to the chest and shoulders. When the shoulder blades become stiff, it stops them from sliding over the upper back in the smooth, fluid way they should, causing them to get stuck. As the shoulders grind against the upper back, the nerves and blood vessels running underneath them become compressed and constricted, causing pain in the surrounding parts of the body to which they are connected. In summary, many of the aches and pains you experience in your chest may have their root cause in stiffness in your shoulder blades.

# SECRET TAKEAWAYS

If you have dull pain around your shoulder blade, or hear a snapping sound when you move your shoulder, and nothing you do to fix the problem seems to work - you probably have severe stiffness around your shoulder blades.

Some of the problems that could stem from a stiff shoulder blade are similar to those caused by a stiff upper back (Secret #4), such as:

- A dull ache and pain around the shoulder blade
- Stooped posture
- Chest twinges
- Shallow breathing, as opposed to deep abdominal breathing
- Aches and discomfort in the upper back
- Pains in shoulders
- Snapping sound when you move your shoulder
- Headaches
- Low energy level, tiredness
- Minimal shoulder movement

Shoulder blade joint stiffness occurs in the upper back and has similar impacts to upper back stiffness. So, in theory, I could just have treated it as an afterthought in one of my upper back secrets. But although my wife Soo's shoulder pain was fixed by relieving the joint stiffness in her upper back, that's not the case with all shoulder pain. Some shoulder pain has roots in the shoulder blade. So you can't always fix it by relaxing the upper back. On top of that, I really wanted to devote one of my secrets to shoulder blade joint stiffness because it's a problem that so many people experience and want solutions for - and it's so painful Despite that, most patients don't realise that the problem is due to their shoulder blades being stiff, and few therapists offer the specialised treatment needed to address the root of the problem. Stretching and strengthening exercises, such as the two I am going to show you below, can help you. But using specialized techniques to directly press on and mobilize stiff shoulder blades offers much more significant and longer lasting benefits. Unfortunately, very few practitioners have any idea of how to do this. Shoulder blades are tough to treat, which takes us back to Mr. Kim. One of the reasons he recently became famous in Korea was that he was one of the only therapists in the world who had come up with a treatment that helped people with painful shoulders caused by stiff shoulder blade joints. As a result of that he's become a very busy man, so hopefully this secret can help those of you with no access to Mr Kim.

# TAKEAWAY EXERCISE

The following two exercises can significantly relieve the pain associated with stiff shoulder blades. Do it daily, repeating 15 times for each exercise to get fast results.

### Scapular wall slides

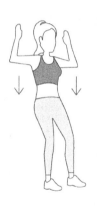 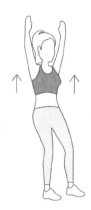

1. Stand with your back against the wall, keeping your feet 15 centimeters away from the wall.
2. With your head, shoulders and elbows against the wall, raise your arms above your head to form a Y position.
3. Bring the arms down. Then up again. Always

keep your head, shoulders and elbows flush against the wall. Keep the repetitions slow and controlled.

*Figure 5.3: The Scapular Wall Slide exercise is designed to move the shoulder blades so the stiffness around the joints becomes loosened*

## Rear delt fly

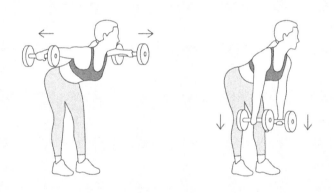

1. Grab two light weights (balls, dumbells or any two objects that are easy to hold and weigh the same) in each hand
2. Bend forward and let your arms hang down
3. Raise your arms to your sides

*Figure 5.4: The Rear Delt Fly exercise uses light weights to help strengthen the muscles that control the shoulder blade movements as well as to loosen the stiffness*

# SORE LEGS? YOUR LOWER BACK IS PROBABLY THE CULPRIT

Have you ever rolled out of bed feeling like you slept on a rock all night? Do you ever try to stand up, only to feel your lower back suddenly buckle? Lower back stiffness is a common problem, that's no secret. According to the WHO, low back pain is the leading single cause of disability in the world (WHO, Musculoskeletal Health, cited above in Secret #2). The problem is, sitting down is really bad for your lower back and maintaining a perfect posture is really hard.

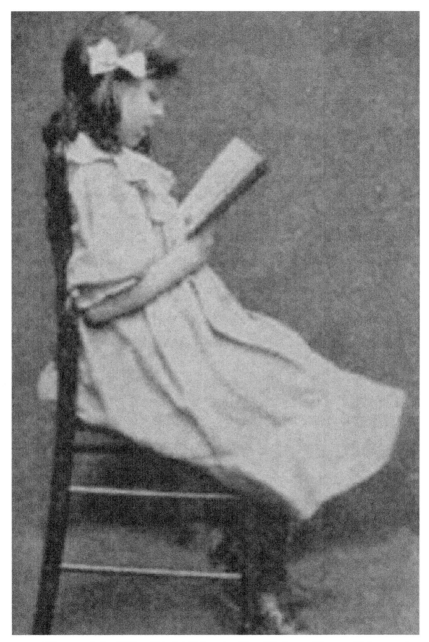

*Figure 6.1: "The Right Way to Read" from Every Woman's Encyclopedia (1910-1912).*

* * *

And even if you do have perfect posture, you're still not immune to the sheer force of gravity. What is a bit of a secret is the great number and variety of leg problems that lower back pain causes, as we shall now see.

Mr. Rowbotham came in to tell me about the severe pain he was feeling just above the back of his ankle, the Achilles tendon. It was so bad that he shouted out in pain when I so much as gently touched him there.

"It's just been getting worse and worse over the last six months. I'm scared to walk on it - I'm afraid the **** thing will completely break down."

We talked some more and he mentioned that the pain was at its worst first thing in the morning when he would get out of bed (which later proved to be an important clue).

Before seeing me, he had spent months trying different treatments. He'd gone for all the usual suspects: calf stretching and strengthening exercises and soft tissue massage directly on his calf and the Achilles tendon. But, unfortunately, none of it worked.

My experience told me that his Achilles tendon problem had reached a chronic stage by now. Because of that, standard stretching and strengthening exercises or soft tissue massage were unlikely to have much of an impact anymore.

It was like putting a bush fire out with a watering can. These standard treatments can be helpful as a part of rehabilitation for Achilles tendonitis, but only in milder cases. And even for such milder cases, it's more effective to address the root cause.

What characterizes standard Achilles heel treatments like stretching and strengthening exercises or soft tissue massage is that they focus directly on the Achilles tendon, or nearby body parts like the calf. Unfortunately, focusing on those areas is a distraction, leading you away from the root cause of the problem. By focusing on them, you miss the wood for the trees.

## Conventional treatments:

Calf Stretches               Achilles Massages

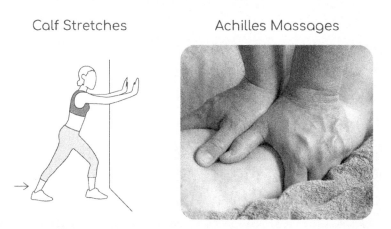

*Figure 6.2: When your Achilles tendon pain is chronic and*

*severe, the conventional approach of massage or stretch exercise offers limited benefits*

I had seen how stiffness in Alex's lower back caused tightness in his thighs. Could it go even further, I wondered, down to the very end of the leg, the Achilles tendon?

There was only one way to find out. I checked his lower back. It was tender when I touched it, displaying a lot of accumulated stiffness and tightness. Mr. Rowbotham had known that he had lower back issues for a while. But they had never seemed severe enough for him to seek treatment, and it had never occurred to him that they might have anything to do with his Achilles tendon problem, for which he very much was seeking treatment - urgently.

It didn't occur to any of the therapists he saw either. This meant he had wasted a lot of time and money on treatments that didn't even stand a chance of dealing with his symptoms, let alone the root cause of his problem.

I can't pretend it was easy to tell him his lower back caused his Achilles heel problem. Mr. Rowbotham had been a history teacher for thirty-six years (in case you're wondering, that's why I call him "Mr Rowbotham" - I still feel strange calling teachers by their first name). He had a way of raising his eyebrows that made you feel as though you hadn't been listening in class.

"My lower back?" He asked this with a thin, weary smile. That put me on the spot and I got a little flustered when I tried to explain. But he was a good teacher, and, after his initial surprise, he helped me get into my stride as I explained the experience with Alex and my other patients.

"The thing is, Sir, I've seen this work. Maybe you should give it a try."

So I went into my usual routine. Repeated mechanical pressure around the joints, focusing on the lower back. I was sure of myself, yet my heart was in my mouth. As I pressed his lower back, I couldn't help looking at his Achilles heel and noticing how far it was from where I was giving him his treatment. His legs were long and they seemed to get longer as I worked.

After some time, I got feedback from Mr Rowbotham that my work on his lower back really was having an impact on his Achilles, but it wasn't much fun to listen to. I was loosening his lower back alright, but that was causing him excruciating pain in his Achilles. He was wincing and groaning, twisting his leg on the table as if I was attacking it with a small pitchfork.

I was actually really pleased. I know a lot of people think we physios do enjoy our patients' suffering but I promise you that's a myth. I wasn't happy that Mr Rowbotham was in pain. I was relieved that the pain he felt in his Achilles while I treated his lower back showed that my intuition about the connection between the two had been correct.

I was able to go on to reassure Mr Rowbotham. The pain he was feeling was something people often feel when they get treatment that goes to the root of their problem. When you go to any manual therapist with a lot of tension, the pressure the therapist applies to loosen your tension hurts at first, as if it was pressing all that tension out. This is called "initial aggravation," of which the saying "it gets worse before it gets better" is a close relative.

In Mr Rowbotham's case, the pain he was feeling was due to the pressure I was applying to his lower back to release the tension there. As that tension reduced, the treatment became less painful. Mr Rowbotham may be blunt, but you couldn't fault his courage. He just grit his teeth and let me keep working on him.

After 30 minutes of treatment, the moment of

truth. I asked him to come off the treatment table and walk around it. I felt like I had won first prize when he gave me an approving nod.

"Well, well. You know, I am finding it much easier to walk. The heel's not as sore. It was painful as h***. And I thought you were pulling the wool over my eyes, but, I have to admit, your idea really works."

When I turned to the literature, I did manage to find a few studies on the relationship between Achilles tendon problems and stiff lower back. A couple of them are helpful: Webborn, 2007 and one by a qualified physiotherapist (Louw, 2019) who practices on patients using this approach. If only I'd been able to quote those studies to Mr. Rowbotham!

My experience with Mr. Rowbotham's Achilles tendon demonstrated that the impact from stiff joints in the lower back travels even farther and has an even wider-ranging impact than with those in the upper back, reaching into the hips and even hamstrings, knees, calf muscles, and ankles.

As a result, stiffness in your lower back can give you the following problems:
- Hip ache
- Tight hamstrings

- Tight calf muscles
- Knee ache
- Achilles tendonitis
- Lack of control in the hips, knees, or ankle joints

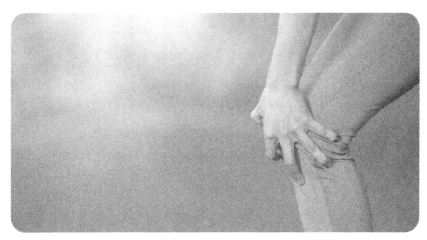

*Figure 6.3: Stiffness in the lower back can cause problems in many parts of the leg. More often than not, the root of the problem lies in the stiff joints in the lower back*

# YOUR "ABS" ARE YOUR ARMOR AGAINST LOWER BACK PAIN

The muscles in our stomach help us digest, that's pretty obvious. What many don't realize, unfortunately, is that those same muscles play an essential role in stabilizing the lower back. If you ever see an advert for a "natural posture brace," what you'll be looking at is a piece of supportive clothing that helps your abdominal muscles hold your lower back in the correct, or "natural," position.

When those muscles are doing their job, they work to support the spine and keep your posture good. That helps a lot to reduce lower back pain (as well as problems like Mr Rowbotham's Achilles). But for that to happen, your core abdominal muscles have to stay strong (Chang et al. 2015).

\* \* \*

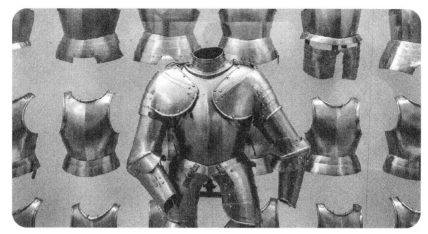

*Figure 6.4: The core muscles in your stomach are a powerful natural "armor" that supports the lower back. They share the loading on the lower back spine. Any lower back treatments need to be accompanied by core strengthening.*

The core muscles work as a brace for the lower back. Imagine you were wearing a tight-fitting suit of metal armor on your body, like a knight in the middle ages.

You would immediately feel that your lower back was well supported. It would be as though the weight on your spine in your lower back had disappeared. Your neighbors might think you were a bit strange, driving to the grocery store in your armor, but your posture would be great.

On the other hand, if your suit of armor was loose and didn't fit you, or if it was made of weak material, it wouldn't provide your lower back with much support, stability or protection. As a result, your lower spine would have to work hard to maintain a good posture, or end up sagging into a poor one. Which would result in lower back pain.

Now try tucking your stomach in so that it's not sticking out. To do that, you need your stomach muscles. If you do that, you will find that your shoulders will tend to draw back and your posture will become straighter. What's happening is that your stomach muscles are doing what the metal armor was doing - it's holding your back straight and taking the weight off the spine. Without drawing strange looks from your neighbors.

That means the secret to reducing lower back pain or avoiding it in the first place is to strengthen those core stomach muscles. The following exercises are designed to do just that.

# TAKEAWAY EXERCISE

## BRIDGE

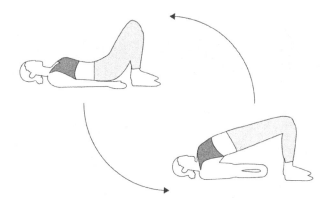

1. Lie on your back with both knees bent.
2. Raise your hips off the floor until your hips are aligned with your knees and shoulders. Hold for 10 seconds.
3. Return to the start position and repeat five times

*Figure 6.5: Bridge exercise strengthens the core muscles, but also works the hamstrings, lower back, and glutes, all of which is essential for treating lower back pain.*

## SEGMENTAL ROTATION

\* \* \*

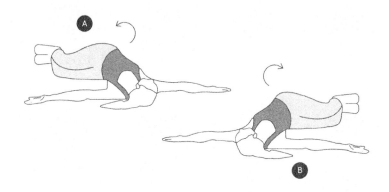

1.  Lie on your back with both knees bent
2.  Keeping your shoulders on the floor, lower your knees slowly to the left, feeling the stretch (A in the picture above) Hold for 10 seconds
3.  Return to the start position. Repeat the exercise to the right (B in the picture above). Repeat 5 times
4.  Make sure you lower your knees slowly, that will make your core muscles work to keep them from dropping too fast.

*Figure 6.6: Segmental rotation is another way to strengthen your core muscles*

# WHY AM I THE ONLY PERSON DOING THIS?

What I don't understand is this. My principle of focusing on joints in the back works in practice. From my experience with countless patients, from Jane to Mr. Rowbotham, I know it works. On top of that, you even find that practical insight backed up in Kendall, the physiotherapist's bible.

Despite that, very few therapists focus on treating stiff joints in the back. Instead, they seem to go for the seemingly obvious, simple solution of massaging the muscles near where their patients feel the pain. Unfortunately, this - very predictably - doesn't deliver lasting benefits to the people suffering pain. Why do they do that, when both theory and practice tell us to do the opposite?

* * *

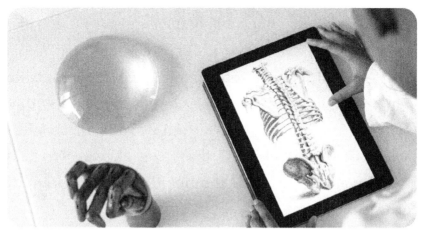

*Figure 6.7: Release of stiff joints is introduced and taught to students at college. But, few therapists use the method extensively simply because it's hard to do physically*

"In theory, there's no difference between theory and practice. In practice, there's a big difference." (Lawrence "Yogi" Berra, baseball player and serial accidental philosopher)

The more I practiced my technique (or what I thought was my technique) of loosening stiff joints in my patients' backs, the more it worked. The more it worked, the more I wondered, "why am I the only physio I know who does this?"

I think there are a few simple reasons. Readers who remember my struggle to find the strength to massage my wife Soo's shoulders after my long daily shift at the physio clinic will probably have guessed it. It's just such hard, repetitive work. It's not something that's easy to admit to, but a lot of people just don't have the stamina or willpower to spend so many hours, day after day, performing this arduous, dull, mechanical task. I can sympathize. I think we all can. No one would want to put their thumbs through this kind of torture.

There's another, albeit less important, reason I think, which readers who followed my treatment of Jane will perhaps suspect. My joint stiffness treatment, although effective, looked really basic, unimpressive. It wasn't something you could really show off.

By contrast, the physio treatments targeted directly at the muscles, although not very effective, look really impressive. As there are many muscles and muscle groups in every part of the body, such treatments can target many different muscles in many different ways and therefore there is an impressive variety to them. They often involve intricate-looking techniques. After the session, the patient can tell a good story about the really original treatment they received. Compared to that, my treatment looks like the ugly duckling. But we know that the ugly duckling turns into a swan. Similarly, joint de-stiffening can transform long-suffering patients into happy, healthy individuals living free from pain.

## Hamstring Stretches

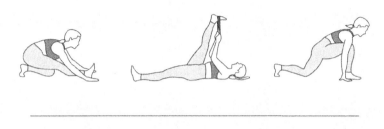

---

## Joint De-Stiffening

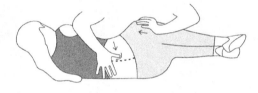

*Figure 6.8: Treatments targeting muscles are often very specific and consist of an impressive variety of techniques, looking impressive, whereas joint releasing treatment in the back looks simple and boring*

# WHY ARE THERE NO OTHER BOOKS OUT THERE SAYING  JOINT DE-STIFFENING IS THE SOLUTION?

If joint de-stiffening is so effective but almost no one is doing it, why has no one written a book about it yet? The short answer is, joint de-stiffening is an established treatment principle, but nobody has fully joined the dots up to now.

Academically speaking, the layperson's term for 'de-stiffening joints' is called 'joint mobilization' (Chiarello 2007). There is clear evidence of the effectiveness of de-stiffening joints in studies.

Many of those studies look at the impact of joint de-stiffening on pain. That impact is significant for the neck (Lee and Lee (no relation), 2017) and for the lower back (Shah and Kage, 2016), for example.

On top of that, the gold standard textbook for manual physiotherapy, Vertebral Manipulation by Geoffrey Maitland (Maitland, 1977) consists almost entirely of de-stiffening techniques targeted at the joint in the back. You'll notice that both of the studies referred to above investigate the impact of "Maitland mobilization" - which in itself shows his status (a search for "Maitland mobilization" on Google Scholar results in around 11,500 references at time of writing). Just by looking at the examination below, you can see that he is examining and treating the joints in the back. For example, he mentions here that it is a joint being examined, but only in passing (page 315).

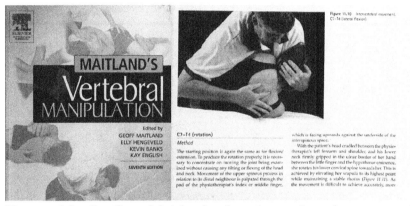

*Figure 6.9: Geoffrey Maitland, the giant of modern manual physiotherapy, tests joint stiffness in the back, and subsequently offers joint de-stiffening treatment to relieve pain in the neck*

In another example, below, he describes a joint de-stiffening procedure in which the therapist places his thumbs on the patient's back. This is exactly what I did in all of the case studies so far. In summary, Maitland, the manual physiotherapy guru, systematically teaches joint de-stiffening work to treat various forms of pain and physical symptoms.

\* \* \*

## EXAMINATION AND TREATMENT TECHNIQUES

### MOBILIZATION

#### Postero–anterior central vertebral pressure (‡)

*Starting position*

The patient lies prone, either with his forehead resting on the backs of his hands or with his head comfortably turned to one side and his arms lying by his sides on the couch. The position depends on the amount of chest tightness created by the 'arms up' position, which is usually reserved for upper thoracic mobilization.

If the patient is on a low couch, the physiotherapist's position for mobilizing the upper thoracic spine (approximately T1–5) needs to be at the head of the patient with her shoulders over the area to be mobilized to enable the direction of the pressure to be at right angles to the surface of the body. The pads of the thumbs are placed on the spinous process, pointing transversely across the vertebral column, and the fingers of each hand are spread out over the posterior chest wall to give stability to the thumbs. As the spinous processes are large, the thumbs may be positioned tip to tip or with the tips side by side in contact with the upper and lower margins of the same spinous process. To gain the best control and feel of movement with the least discomfort to the patient, the pressure should be transmitted through the thumbs so that the interphalangeal joints are hyperextended. This enables the softest part of the pad to be flat over the spinous processes, with a slight degree of flexion in the metacarpophalangeal joints. Not only is this more comfortable for the patient, but it hinders the physiotherapist's intrinsic muscles from producing the pressure.

above may be used, but the essential factor is that the direction of the pressure must be at right angles to the body surface at the level. This means that the shoulders may need to be anywhere between vertically above the lower thoracic spine and vertically above the sacrum (*Figure 11.14*). If the patient has difficulty lying prone because extension is painful, a small pillow under the chest will assist. The physiotherapist's position must also allow pressure to be applied to the spinous process using the anteromedial aspect of the fifth metacarpal, similar to that described on pages 370–371 for the lumbar spine. However, it may be essential to avoid direct contact between the pisiform and the spinous process for the sake of comfort (*Figure 11.14*).

#### Method

The mobilizing is carried out by an oscillating pressure on the spinous processes, produced by the body and transmitted through the arms to the thumbs. It is important that this pressure is applied by the body weight over the hands and not by a squeezing action with the thumbs themselves. The fingers, which are spread out over the patient's back, should not exert any pressure but act only as stabilizers for the thumbs. It is easy to dissipate the pressure and lose the effectiveness of the thumbs by faulty use of the fingers.

If the physiotherapist's elbows are kept slightly flexed and the thumbs maintained in the position of hyperextension of interphalangeal joints and slight flexion of metacarpophalangeal joints, the pressure can be transmitted to the pads of the thumbs through this series of strong springs. This springing action at the joints can readily be seen as the body weight is applied during the mobilizing.

*Figure 6.10: Maitland goes into detail to show how joint de-stiffening treatment is performed on various parts of the neck and back. His approach is widely taught as an integral part of all physio courses across the globe*

The benefits of joint de-stiffening on pain are well established, and the treatment technique is taught as an integral part of all physio courses in the UK and globally. It's also part of the "know how" that extends beyond classic textbooks like Maitland. However, there are a few reasons why these studies and textbooks don't quite join the dots:

\* \* \*

1.  Most manual therapists know that joint de-stiffening is the most effective form of manual treatment, and they take it for granted, to the point that they don't see any reason to explain the point to their patients. Therefore, the knowledge and information about joint de-stiffening tends to be kept within that small group of insiders.

2.  Knowing that joint de-stiffening works doesn't get professional therapists very far, because they can't do much with the information. It's too hard for a human therapist to do. Indeed, Maitland only recommends performing joint de-stiffening for a minute at a time because - as a practitioner - he was aware of how hard it is.

3.  As a result, joint de-stiffening is very rarely practiced and, when practiced, only in short stretches because it's so hard and also boring, unglamorous. This helps keep the subject of joint mobilization relatively obscure.

4.  People outside the manual therapy profession assume that muscle massage is the best (or even only) available option for them, because that's mostly what they get.

\* \* \*

In summary, it does seem strange that I was the first person to treat Mr Rowbotham's Achilles by loosening the joints in his back, but when you look back across the way treatment has developed it makes a lot of sense. Not a lot of research is done into physiotherapy, most of the knowledge is passed on as knowhow.

The little research we do have recognizes that there is a link between joint stiffness and muscles, but gets the cause and effect the wrong way around. It also understands that stiff joints can stretch nerves—and Kendall's physio bible emphatically states that all mechanical pain is derived from stretched nerves - but none of the literature puts two and two together. In other words, the idea that most mechanical pain is caused by stiff joints is based on well-established principles which have been lying scattered through a variety of separate, almost self-contained pieces of research and practical manuals. My method is based on those well-established principles and so I can't really say I am inventing something entirely new in this book. What I think this book does for the first time is draw these different principles together into a unified theory.

The thing is, people like Maitland and Kendall write textbooks to help physios do their jobs well. They're not trying to win research awards. So when Maitland's book consists almost entirely of joint loosening exercises, you don't find him writing "How interesting, all the exercises in this book mobilize joints." That's probably because it's obvious to Maitland, so obvious he doesn't notice it. And it's definitely because that theoretical observation doesn't help the book achieve its aim - to teach physiotherapists good physiotherapy techniques.

Even though the theory isn't developed, a core of experienced practitioners knows that you can help muscle pain by de-stiffening joints in the back. But that doesn't make much of an impact, because, even though they know this, physios are only human and implementing joint de-stiffening is hard labor for which they will gain few plaudits.

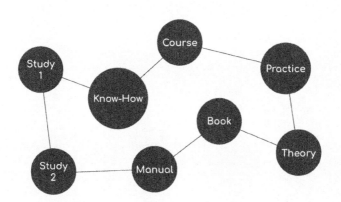

*Figure 6.11: 'Joint de-stiffening' has been practiced for a long time, individual descriptions and studies of it are scattered*

*around here and there and it's hard to understand the principles that underlie them. They only start to make sense when put together*

I hope this book finally joins the dots, showing how the many common presentations which are treated with muscle massage - day to day by millions of therapists, without ever making it into any academic study - are best treated by joint de-stiffening.

# PARKINSON'S DISEASE AND STIFF BACK

This section is in memory of my late, dear friend Mr Davies.

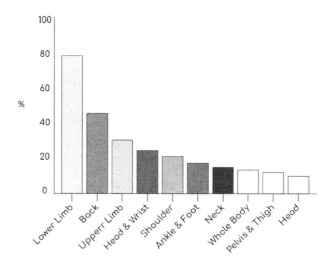

*Figure 7.1: back pain and leg pain are very common in patients diagnosed with Parksinson's Disease. The muscles in Parkinson's become tight, and joints get stiff due to lack of dopamine hormone release. Graph from Li et al, 2022*

One of the most common physical characteristics of patients living with Parkinson's Disease (PD) is that their back is tight and the joints in their back are stiff. As a result, PD patients often suffer from pain in their back and legs (Li et al., 2022). This is due to a lack of dopamine hormone release, which, according to consensus (including Parkinson's UK), is responsible for the general difficulty people living with Parkinson's experience with movement in general.

Taking drugs that induce or stimulate the production of dopamine, such as Levodopa, helps people manage their Parkinson's condition. Another common way for people living with Parkinson's to help their symptoms is regular exercise classes and physiotherapy, which helps them alleviate their pain and improve their movement.

I have had many opportunities to work with people living with Parkinson's while practicing as a physio. As well as their physical symptoms, I noticed one particularly interesting thing about people who live with Parkinson's, which doesn't fit the stereotype. Many of them were socio-economically successful; a lot of them were successful accountants, lawyers and business people. They were often articulate speakers and writers, incisive and impressive. I was curious whether anyone else had noticed this and looked to see if I could find any research on things like the income or professional outcomes of people living with PD, but I couldn't find any academic studies that supported what I had observed, although I did find one publication that shared my observation (Luca A, et al, 2019). So I can't be sure whether what I observed is a real phenomenon or just a coincidence among the relatively small sample of people living with PD whom I treated. Whatever the science eventually decides, there's no doubt that I really enjoyed the time I spent with my patients living with Parkinson's.

When Mr Davies, who was born in 1939 like my friend Kerry Napuk (to whom this book is dedicated), visited my clinic for the first time, he presented like my other PD patients, both physically and in his personality. He was organized, had impressive problem solving skills, and had worked as Managing Director for an international manufacturing company for many years, including a long stint in China. He had enjoyed his time in China and built close relationships with many of his Chinese colleagues and neighbors. He was cosmopolitan, open minded, with a good sense of humor. I liked him..

It didn't take long for us to become good friends. For our regular monthly get together we would go out for a traditional fish & chips lunch in Edinburgh Scotland, where we both lived. I hadn't heard of "fish n' chips" before I came to the UK and you may not have had the pleasure. Although the UK is good at a lot of things, most people wouldn't immediately include British cooking among them (that may be slowly changing with celebrity chefs like Nigella Lawson, Gordon Ramsay, Jamie Oliver or Heston

Blumenthal). As a result, for a long time the most popular dishes ordered in British restaurants tended to be based on recipes from other countries, mainly India, China and Italy (with notable adaptations, like the Scottish deep fried pizza). But fish & chips is a popular dish that is also a British cultural icon. It's basically french fries and deep fried, battered fish (usually cod or haddock).. It's so popular that you find a lot of British families going for a "fish supper" (as they say in Scotland) once a week.

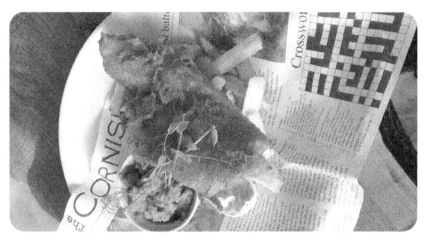

*Figure 7.2: Potatoes and fish are deep fried in oil to produce tasty fish & chips, which is regarded by many as the most popular dish in the UK*

Apologies if you've heard about fish and chips before. It's a subject close to my heart because it reminds me of discovering the UK when I moved there to study physiotherapy, and of my conversations with Mr Davies. We would talk about a lot of different things, swapping stories about places we'd been and the people we met there. I had thought of a new product I wanted to develop and was thinking of taking the plunge as an entrepreneur, and he was very generous with his advice, having overseen quite a few product launches during his career.. Mr Davies also wrote poetry (poets are an unusual breed in the world of international manufacturing) which he would show me and which I liked very much. He also edited his church's bi-monthly magazine, of which he would hand me a copy when he came for his regular physio sessions at my clinic.

Like other people living with Parkinson's, Mr Davies had very tight joints and muscles in his back and neck. They really restricted his ability to move, particularly his walking. Following my now well established technique, I would spend about 30 minutes releasing joint stiffness in his back with my two thumbs. The treatment had the desired outcome, giving him immediate (albeit partial) relief to his back pain, and helping him walk better with longer steps and a more fluent motion. He would come every other week, but that still wasn't enough for him. In an ideal world, he would have liked to have me practice my treatment on him every day, which wasn't a possibility; even though he was successful, he hadn't reached the stage where he could afford his own live-in physio.

Despite his PD, Mr Davies was very active - a regular angler and a weekly golf player, as well as his poetry, editing and church attendance. He did what he enjoyed, using both his mind and his body actively, was generous with his time and a good natured and positive person, who never complained about anything.

Later, when I was testing an early version of the back therapy machine on which I had asked for his advice, Mr Davies was one of the first to volunteer. He was very encouraging about the machine's potential, saying he could move and walk better after he had a session on it.

Sadly, Mr Davies passed away during the Covid-19 pandemic. I was never able to let him try the latest version of our product, which he had helped me develop and promised to offer the live-in physio he wished he had. The most sad thing of all was that I couldn't say goodbye to him or attend his funeral, due to the strict COVID-19 restrictions that were in place at the time. When I spoke to his widow on the phone, I could tell how much she had loved him and how much she missed him. He really was an amazing guy and I miss him too.

# PATIENTS WITH PARKINSON'S AND OTHER NEUROLOGICAL CONDITIONS HAVE VERY STIFF BACKS

My experience of the stiff backs my Parkinson's patients presented with was consistent with a broader observation that (unlike my experience of the professional success of people with Parkinson's) can be found in the scientific literature, stiff backs are also highly prevalent among people suffering a wide variety of chronic health issues, particularly those with neurological issues.

One of the explanations that have been advanced for this in the literature is that people living with chronic pain or neurological conditions tend to spend more time at home and move and walk less, leaving them with tight muscles and stiff joints (Nimwegen et al. 2011).

That's why, unsurprisingly, many health bodies recommend regular movement and physical activity as strategies to improve the physical and mental wellbeing of people with chronic health conditions (see for example the UK's NICE Guidelines, 2017)

It does seem as though regularly releasing the stiff joints in their neck and back really helps people with neurological conditions, as much if not more than the other conditions I treat in patients, reducing not just pain in the back but in the legs too and, above all, helping them move better. Ultimately, it was an enhanced version of this that Mr Davies was hoping for when he wanted me to treat him every day.

# ONLY TREATING THE BODY IS OFTEN NOT ENOUGH

My experience with Mr Davies and other patients with neurological conditions illustrates a fundamental point about therapy in general, not just back therapy, with which I would like to finish this section.

From time to time I come across eye-catching news headlines about promising medical treatments undergoing clinical trials. Those headlines raise people's hopes that - if the trials are successful - the featured treatment might eradicate certain diseases like various cancers, Multiple Sclerosis (MS) or Parkinson's disease (PD). Unfortunately, after around two decades of reading those headlines, my observation is that the treatments don't live up to the hype.

Despite that, these headlines are exciting for the patients and their family. All too often though, after a few years the hype dies down and the story gets forgotten, while the press latches on to the latest promising treatment, and so the cycle continues. This is not to cast shade on the research. It just shows how difficult it is to create a really effective medical treatment for chronic conditions for human beings. What is really noticeable is that the human body just doesn't respond to treatment like that of a mouse in a lab.

Images of headline news 'Cancer cure finally found' "Newly trialed miracle treatment could change the lives of those with MS' 'When will there be a cure for Rheumatoid Arthritis'?

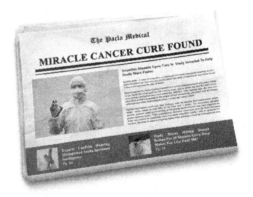

*Figure 7.3: I have observed many 'miracle treatment' headlines in the media over decades, but almost none lived up to the hype. It shows the challenges we face when dealing with human body and mind*

\* \* \*

Having observed many of those sensationalist headlines over the years, I have become a little cynical about what people are selling. I'm suspicious of any news story claiming a 'miracle cure' for chronic conditions, including cancer, MS, Parkinson's, Rheumatoid Arthritis or dementia. There is a fundamental reason for my caution, which goes beyond my disappointment with any particular "new treatment" newsflash that didn't live up to expectations.

My reason is this: the human body and mind are inseparable, and human health is the result of a complex interaction between physiology and psychology (Ohrnberger et al. 2017). The 'psychological' part makes predicting the impact of any treatment on human health very difficult. That makes it very hard to find a miracle cure for us humans. It's also why identical treatments often produce very different results for two different people with exactly the same condition. The mental, emotional, 'psychological' part of the equation plays a big role in our health, but that role is exceptionally difficult to predict or influence.

# TEACH YOUR BODY TO FISH

My observation of the close connection between mind and body while treating patients has given me the profound conviction that any external intervention, including my own manual treatment, should aim to help the body restore its own self-healing ability. The body isn't a machine. That means there isn't something outside of our body - a drug, a massage, a brace or whatever - that can completely heal it the way you would fix a car or a dishwasher. It's like the saying 'heaven helps those who help themselves.' Any external cure or fix can only be truly effective if it teaches or stimulates the body to heal itself. And that can only happen if the body and mind are working together in harmony.

Often, the best way to enable the body to overcome chronic pain, injury or illness is to reboot or strengthen its immune system. One of the things I have consistently observed is that the most successful treatments are those that help the body produce healing hormones like serotonin, melatonin and dopamine. I'm convinced one of the main reasons loosening joints in the back is so effective is that it stimulates those beneficial hormones. If we take care of our body well, it will produce a healthy quantity of those healing hormones on its own and maintain itself in a state of healthy balance - a state doctors call "homeostasis."

The best external therapies encourage our bodies to heal themselves and keep themselves in homeostasis. Our bodies are incredible, the result of hundreds of thousands of years of evolution across hundreds of trillions of human beings. A lot of that good work has been spoiled by modern developments like sedentary lifestyles or excessive consumption of processed food (this framework was crystalized for me by reading an amazing book called Anti-Fragile, by the celebrated options trader, probability theorist and "flaneur," Nassim Taleb). The best therapies aim to put things back into balance, so that this beautifully created and evolved human body functions the way it was designed to - which is the best way.

That's why getting enough good quality sleep is so important. That's why loving relationships with your family and friends are so important. That's why eating healthily, meditating and taking regular exercise can be as powerful as any medication. All of them work in the same way as the best external treatments. They create a relaxing harmony between your body and mind and encourage the production of healthy serotonin, melatonin and dopamine hormones, so your body can stay healthy using its own resources, its own energy. The well-known East African saying, "Give someone a fish, you feed them for a day. If you teach them how to fish, you feed them for a lifetime" applies here. Giving people drugs and other forms of external interventions can keep them healthy for a day. By teaching their body to produce its own beneficial hormones, there's a good chance they'll stay healthy for a lifetime.

Secrets #3-#7 introduce a framework that I have developed from my physiotherapy practice, research, textbooks and practitioner knowhow. That framework is there to help you look beyond the obvious. It tells you not to focus on the part of your body in which you feel the pain, whether that's your elbow or your ankle. You can use that framework to find the part of your body that is the root cause of your pain. That part could be anywhere from your neck to your lower back joints.

The following two sections have a different emphasis. They will reveal two lifestyle principles that you can use to stay healthy and which I recommend to my patients. But they still follow the same fundamental principle - look for the root causes of the problem, don't be distracted by where the symptoms are.

# SECTION THREE

"A change in bad habits leads to a change in life."

—Jenny Craig

# DON'T BE A SITTING DUCK

There are a couple of stories in this section which I'm kind of embarrassed to share with you. Both basically involve me not practicing what I preach as a physiotherapist and paying the price.

A few years ago, Peter, a colleague of mine, and I were lifting a heavy box together. We were maneuvering in a tight spot and I ended up twisting myself into an awkward position. I felt a twinge as we lifted the box, but it was only when I got home that I realized I had really hurt my lower back (the lumbosacral joint to be precise). I had just turned 40 that year. Since then, that part of my back has never been the same. Especially if I sit for long hours without a break, my back tells me it's not happy and I need to stand up!

Us physios are human like the rest. We make the same mistakes that force other people to come to us for help. We don't always have perfect posture (that's ballet you're thinking of). So don't be too hard on yourself if your posture hasn't always been great. The key is what you do about it from now on.

People have to remember that after they turn 40, their muscle mass decreases at almost 1% each year (Volpi et al. 2004). Muscles act as a kind of scaffold for your back, supporting it and absorbing the weight, just as abdominal muscles support your lower back (as we saw in Secret #6). The reduced muscle mass encouraged by aging means that scaffolding gets weaker and gives your back less support. Prolonged sitting accelerates this process.

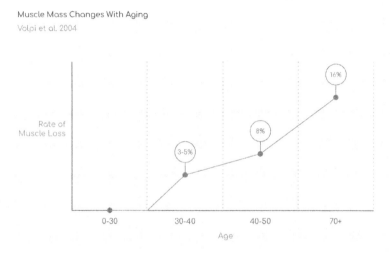

Muscle Mass Changes With Aging
Volpi et al. 2004

*Figure 8.1: After we turn 30, we naturally lose muscle mass unless we compensate with strengthening exercises. The loss of muscle mass, unfortunately, accelerates after we turn 40 and keeps accelerating in every subsequent decade.*

After I learned that my body was shedding those precious muscles at a rate of almost 1% every year, I started doing everything I could to compensate for that loss, which means regular strengthening exercises. Nothing fancy - I do plank, bridging, squatting and push-ups a few times a week.

# EXERCISES USING YOUR OWN BODY WEIGHT ARE THE MOST NATURAL WAY OF STRENGTHENING YOUR MUSCLES

A lot of people think strengthening exercises are for body builders or gym rats. That's so wrong. Building up your muscles and your strength is a key part of keeping your whole body healthy and staying free from injury.

The good news is that it only takes a few simple exercise routines to achieve the goal of drastically reducing the rate of age-related muscle loss. All you need is two days a week of muscle strengthening activity (Physical Activity Guidelines for Americans 2nd edition, 2018).

You don't even need any fancy, expensive equipment. The weight of your body is enough, although a pair of dumbbells can be helpful too. What you do need is some creativity to get those major muscles (legs, hips, back, abdomen, chest, shoulders, and arms) strong. All you need to do is choose just two to three exercises and invest only 20 minutes at a time, twice a week.

\* \* \*

Here are examples of exercises I recommend:

- Six push-ups, do 3 sets (i.e. do your six pushups three times)
- Ten triceps dips, do 2 sets
- Fifteen step-ups, do 3 sets
- Fifteen lunges, do 3 sets for each leg
- Ten squats, do 3 sets
- Five chest 1kg dumbbell presses 5 repetitions, do 3 sets
- Five lying 1kg dumbbell flies, do 3 sets
- Ten pullover 1kg dumbbells, do 3 sets

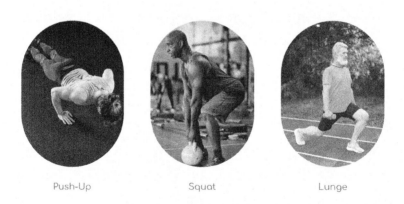

Push-Up          Squat          Lunge

*Figure 8.2: Use your own body weight when doing strengthening exercises. It is the most natural way to strengthen the muscles and doesn't put undue strain on your body.*

Apart from the three dumbbell exercises, all of

these exercises use the weight of your body. And you can do all of them without going to the gym.

Do two of any of those a week and you'll go a long way toward maintaining your strength as you age. You'll be amazed how quickly you notice your body becoming stronger.

A lot of people are self-conscious about their fitness and that can get in the way of building your strength. So I want to share two rules of thumb to help you get over any self-consciousness.

- Number one, it doesn't matter how much exercise you do to start. You just need to start somewhere. If it's just one push up, that's fine. Do one push up.
- Number two, never do less than what you did the last time. So if you did two push ups last time, do at least two this time. The thing is, you know you can do it. You did it last time. And if you keep doing it, you'll build strength. Next time you might say "you know what, I'll do an extra one this time." Before you know it, you'll be doing ten, twenty, thirty … As long as you don't go backwards, who knows how far you can go?

\* \* \*

That's an example of me practicing what I preach. Unfortunately, there is one glaring counter-example I have to own up to. The worst thing about it is that I failed to follow one of the precepts I preached about the loudest to my patients.

# A HARD DAY AT THE OFFICE GETS EVEN HARDER

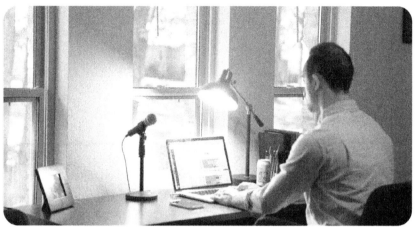

*Figure 8.3: Sitting is the new 'smoking' (Levine 2014). Repeated prolonged sitting is the number one culprit of neck and back stiffness*

The day started like any other day. I was working at my desk. I had stopped practicing as a physio to work full time on launching a therapy robot that would do the work for me (described further below in Secret #9). But it soon became a very memorable, unusual day for all the wrong reasons.

I started to feel an ache creeping up my right shoulder. The pain became so intense that I couldn't continue to work anymore. I just had to stop.

I went straight into physio mode, except this time the patient was me. I stood up and started doing shoulder stretches. They helped, but I was still curious.

What had caused this sudden pain in my shoulder?

My physio brain went through the checklist. Accidents? Negative.

Sports? Nothing to report.

Bumps, collisions? Nothing.

I couldn't figure it out.

Now I was like a dog hunting for a rat. I was on high alert for anything which might lead me to the source of the pain.

As the day progressed, my shoulder ache wasn't constant. Instead, it would get worse, and then it would get better. And the pattern was clear.

If I was sitting down, whether working at my desk or relaxing on the sofa, the ache would worsen. On the other hand, if I stood up or walked around it would ease up a little.

So I tried to rest my shoulders on the back of the couch.

I even tried to rest my elbows on the arm of my desk chair.

Sadly none of that made much difference.

The only thing that helped was lying down with my shoulder placed on the bed or the sofa.

But lying down all day wasn't an option.

I needed to work.

People standing to work was no longer unusual by now and many forward thinking companies were introducing standing desks, but lying down to work was a step too far.

Adjusting my position, lying down - I was sure that was just dealing with the symptoms. So I paused my work and went for a walk.

Like many of you, stepping away and taking a break lets me get some perspective and allows my brain to work out in the background, looking for solutions.

It was a typical Edinburgh day. The wind was blowing. The city was covered by a white sea-mist locals call "the haar," which made everything look mysterious and spooky. The author Robert Louis Stevenson based his famous story "The strange case of Dr. Jekyll and Mr. Hyde" (1886) in Edinburgh, and it was one of those days when you wouldn't have been surprised to see Mr. Hyde dart out from one of the courtyards I walked past.

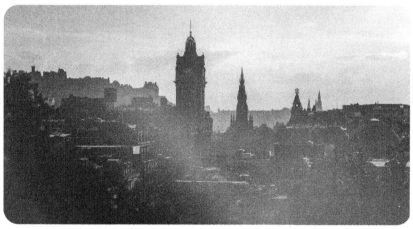

*Figure 8.4: Edinburgh lies on the southern shore of the sea. When warm air moves over the cooler water, it causes moisture in the air to condense and form the "haar," which is then blown*

*inland by the wind creating this gloomy, atmospheric mist.*

Although the haar got heavier and wetter as I walked, the mist in my mind slowly cleared. I noticed that my neck and upper back were very stiff, and that was undoubtedly because I had spent most of the last few days bending forward to look at my computer screen. The pain in my shoulder wasn't due to anything I'd done to my shoulder. Instead, it was due to the stiffness in my upper back and neck joints, affecting the nerves and blood vessels that bring vital fluids and sensory information to my shoulder (as described above in Secret #4).

# SITTING IS THE NUMBER ONE CULPRIT
# FOR A STIFF NECK AND BACK.

If you sit all day, you're putting your health at risk every day. That may sound dramatic, but I'm afraid it's true. If you have a demanding or stressful office job, your back is doing a lot of work to keep you in a sitting position. Even worse, you often end up slouching as you forget to sit straight (which is why keeping those core abs strong is so important, see Secret #6).

You also tense up as you peer at a line of code or a key clause in a contract. Your head bends to read an important message from a colleague on Slack. Your shoulders and arms are busy clicking on "Save" or selecting options on a supplier's website. It isn't good for you, whatever you're doing while you're sitting.

\* \* \*

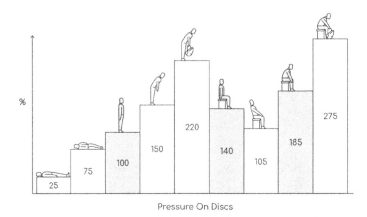

Pressure On Discs

*Figure 8.5: If standing straight is the baseline (100), slouch-sitting increases the stress on your back to 185, almost double the stress of standing.*

Sitting stiffens our neck and back twice as much as walking (Ebfraheim. M.D. 2010). 30 minutes of sitting is often regarded as the tipping point (Rutten et al. 2013), after which your neck and back start to get stiff enough to cause you trouble.

# REVERSE-ENGINEERING THE CAUSE OF YOUR PAIN

So we know prolonged sitting stiffens the neck and back, which is both painful and unhealthy. Because sitting is so bad for you, I want to show you how to "reverse-engineer" what happens to you when you sit, to unpick the mechanism that's causing you pain. Using the reverse-engineering technique I'm about to show you, you will be able to figure out whether the pain you're experiencing - be it in your head, back, shoulders, arms, legs or feet - is really due to your stiff back, or caused by something else.

For example, let's say you have pain in your right knee. Next, imagine you're trying to figure out where exactly it's coming from. You try a foam roller, or strengthening exercises for your quadriceps, hamstring or glutes - but none of them make a difference. You keep doing those exercises for a week, but you still feel the pain. You haven't had any accidents, falls, sports injuries or anything else that seems like an obvious reason for your knee pain. And standing or walking makes your knee painful or heavy.

Time for some reverse-engineering. First, if you're going to sit down, consider how sore your knee is before you're sitting down and then check again one hour later (you may want to use a timer): is your knee pain worse AFTER you've been sitting for an hour or more? Or is there no noticeable difference? You may want to keep a note of this.

Next, keep observing the relationship between how much knee pain you're suffering and how much time you're spending sitting from day to day. You may want to keep a record of your subjective pain score on different days (for example, you might score your knee pain at 2/10 on Wednesday and 8/10 on Thursday) and how long you've been sitting on each day (for example, three hours on Wednesday, eight hours on Thursday).

Now, if:

    a.   Your knee pain is worse after you spend an hour or more sitting

    b.   Your knee pain is worse on any given day if you spent longer sitting on that day

then it's probably due to joint stiffness in your back, especially the lower back on the same side as the knee that's giving you pain.

As I explained in this section, the reason for this simple connection is that sitting down makes the joints in your lower back go stiff. Those stiff joints then put pressure on the nerves (and fasciae) that travel to the knee. It's the pressure on those nerves (and fasciae) that is causing your knee pain.

This reverse-engineering technique works for any part of your body. If the particular pain you experience in a particular part of your body gets worse after you spend a while sitting, that pain is probably caused by joint stiffness somewhere in your back. This simple technique won't turn you into a clinician, but it's an easy, common sense rule of thumb that's easy to pick up and can save you a lot of time and money.

# BREAK UP YOUR SITTING CYCLE EVERY 30 MINUTES

Now I'd be surprised if I was the first person to tell you that sitting for too long isn't good for you. That's well known, although most people are taken aback when they discover that sitting puts almost twice as much strain on your back as standing. I hope my own sore shoulder case study offered a salutary example of the far-reaching problems caused by sitting too long and making your upper back stiffen up.

So if you have a sedentary job or lifestyle, it's essential to make an effort to move around as much as possible. Even small changes can make a big difference.

I also want to offer some solutions. These are well known, but it's surprising how many people don't use them:

\* \* \*

## Breaking The Sitting Cycle

1. Set the alarm for every 30 minutes on your smartphone.

2. Every time the alarm goes off, just stand up for as little as 10 seconds, stretching your body or even walking about. Try to look out of the window or into the distance to help your eyes rest.

3. Take a brisk walk during your lunch break

4. Try to get moving whenever you can.

*Figure 8.6: Breaking the sitting cycle every 30 minutes is often enough to prevent the development of severe stiffness in your back.*

If you suffer from chronic pain, you may be tempted to stay in one position all day to avoid aggravating your symptoms. This may involve sitting all day. However, that can do more harm than good. As we've seen, prolonged sitting can lead to several problems, including muscle stiffness, poor circulation and increased pain.

You may not have implemented the alarm-on-your-phone solution because you're not tech-savvy. If so, I would just ask one of your friends or family for advice, they will help you find an easy way to use a timer to stop you from sitting for too long.

Now you know how severe and far-reaching the impact of back stiffness is. I hope that will encourage you to adopt this easy solution to stop you from sitting down too long. It's not a very sophisticated solution. But it's incredibly effective. The key is to do it. That will do wonders for your neck and back and for your health in general.

# KEEP THOSE
# SHOULDERS MOVING

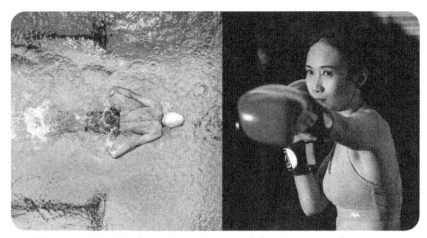

*Figure 9.1: Both swimming and boxing involve constant shoulder movements, and are hugely effective for releasing the joint stiffness built around the neck and back*

What do swimming and boxing have in common?

The two are very different. No one swims with boxing gloves or boxes with flippers. But both have one thing in common: they force you to constantly move your shoulders.

Over the years, I have found that frequent or regular shoulder motion is a really potent activity, although it may not seem like you're achieving much while you're doing it. That's because it's tremendously effective for releasing the stiffness in both your neck and your back joints.

That constant shoulder movement "chips away" at the stiffness in your neck and back. Do it long enough, and you'll feel the difference. Remember, we saw in all the Secrets in this book related to stiff upper back and neck that those can cause you a lot of trouble. So it's easy to see that chipping that stiffness away with constant shoulder motion will do you a lot of good.

But constantly moving your shoulders isn't natural. The beauty of both boxing and swimming is that they more or less force you to do it. If you're in deep enough water, you have to keep moving your shoulders if you don't want to drown. While in the ring, if you keep your shoulders still, you're asking to get knocked out.

Swimming is known to be an excellent workout for your whole body, but did you ever actually consider that it can also be particularly beneficial for your back?

In fact, if you're suffering from back pain, swimming is an excellent, low-impact way to loosen your back up.

Boxing is just as good if that is more of your thing - as long as you avoid getting a black eye in the process.

Of course, exercise in general is good, and the most important thing is to find a form of exercise you enjoy. But if you want to work those stiff joints, boxing (or boxing training if you don't want to get in the ring) and swimming are hard to beat.

I'm not much of a dancer, but dancing,

especially rhythmic dances like Salsa or Merengue, involve a lot of shoulder movement. If you're really feeling the beat, your shoulders will start moving naturally. So if you don't like contact sports or are afraid of the water, dancing is a good alternative. It's also fun and sociable.

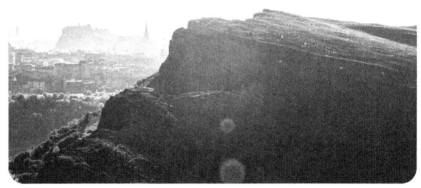

*Figure 9.2: I often go for a run around Holyrood Park and Arthur's Seat in Edinburgh, Scotland. One full circle is about 5.5 km. It's hilly, with spectacular views that make the experience even more enjoyable*

I like to run around Holyrood Park and Arthur's Seat, both well-known Edinburgh landmarks. I usually run for about 40 minutes. I do about three and a half miles (5.5km) in that time. Afterwards, the good feeling in my back can last for around two days. It really helps compensate for all that sitting at the desk.

Going back to the shoulders, I make sure to swing my arms back and forth constantly while I run, so all of the joints in my neck, shoulder blades, upper and lower back get moved about during the running. Doing that helps me exercise my whole body, and if you get it right, it can give your running time a good rhythm.

But if I had to pick one of those activities, it would be swimming. It requires many different shoulder motions. When you swim, your shoulders rotate clockwise and counter-clockwise, combining internal and external rotation, and the shoulder blades move forwards and backward. No other exercise offers the variety of shoulder motion that swimming does. That's why it's the best of all exercises to keep your shoulders moving, in my humble opinion.

# THE BEST EXERCISES FOR RELEASING BACK STIFFNESS

- Swimming
- Boxing
- Dancing
- Jogging

*Figure 9.3: Whatever exercise you do, make sure your shoulders move about!*

# SECTION FOUR

"I never did anything by accident, nor did any of my inventions come by accident; they came by work."

—Thomas A. Edison

# GET YOUR OWN LIVE-IN THERAPIST

(It's Easier Than You'd Think)

"OK, Gillian, have you downloaded the App?"

"I have, I have Chongsu," Gillian laughed.

It was hard to say which of us was most in suspense, but I'm sure it was me.

"Are you ready, Gillian?"

"I'm ready, Chongsu."

After that, for me, there was no going back. No escape. No off-ramp. No excuses. Either this thing was going to work, or I was done.

Gillian had been a patient of mine for a long time. She had lived with Multiple Sclerosis (MS) since the birth of her first child. Although she feels that birth was a blessing that more than compensated, MS is still a great challenge and a real burden for her.

I had worked with many people with MS as a physio. The condition is common in Scotland, where I opened my first clinic. At first, people living with MS would come to see me because their backs were stiff. Later, I realized that nearly everyone with MS presents with back stiffness.

As with nearly all my patients, I used my signature technique of mobilizing the joints in the back and neck of my patients living with MS.

With them, however, something unique happened.

The symptoms of their MS improved.

They had more energy.

They felt less pain.

They could walk better.

They were able to control their bladder better.

All thanks to the positive effects of releasing stiffness in their back.

By coincidence, one of my patients living with MS was an actress called Alison Peebles. She had been acting in the famous Scottish detective series Taggart when MS cut her acting career short - or so it seemed at first. But, after I treated her, she was able to work again. The story was featured in The Sunday Times newspaper. That's when the floodgates opened and people with MS came from hundreds of miles away for my treatment.

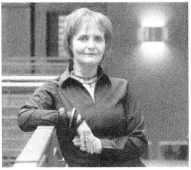

No.9/805  JULY 28, 2013                    £2.90 | £2 TO SUBSCRIBERS  SCOTLAND

# THE SUNDAY TIMES

**Peebles feared MS would confine her to a wheelchair**

## MS treatment helps actress get back on her feet

**Mark Macaskill**

ONE of Scotland's leading actresses appears to be winning her fight against multiple sclerosis with a revolutionary physiotherapy treatment.

Alison Peebles, whose credits include Taggart, River City, High Times, AfterLife and Sex Traffic, was diagnosed with primary progressive MS — characterised by a steady worsening of symptoms without remission — in 2001.

A decline in her mobility, causing her to collapse frequently, had forced Peebles to prepare for confinement to a wheelchair.

However, she has experienced dramatic improvements in her walking, balance and flexibility after treatment involving gentle manipulation of the spine to release tension.

"The benefits of this treatment have been quite dramatic," said Peebles. "I was collapsing all the time as I had poor balance and strength. I was mentally and physically exhausted.

"Now, after 18 weeks of treatment, my walking, balance and vision are hugely improved and my body is much more flexible. I still use a crutch, but if I continue like this, I feel optimistic that I can keep on my feet and delay the imminent need for a wheelchair.

"I am more supple, I am standing straighter and have more energy."

Peebles has been treated by Chongsu Lee, a physiotherapist and former engineer for Hyundai in South Korea, at his Edinburgh clinic.

The technique involves gentle manipulation of the spine and surrounding soft tissue to release tension from the body, allowing better movements of the neck, shoulders and back.

As tension around the spine gradually eases off, blood and lymph circulation and nerve function improve.

"When Alison came to see me she was walking haltingly, her posture was stooped and she looked quite tired," said Lee. "These symptoms and other issues seemed to have been affecting her quality of life and acting career."

The improvement in Peebles's condition means she can go ahead and direct Bite the Bullet, a play starring Sandy Nelson and Keith Warwick, at the Assembly Rooms as part of the Edinburgh Fringe in August. She recently co-wrote and starred in the National Theatre of Scotland play My Shrinking Life, dramatising her experience of the disease.

Between 100 and 140 people in every 100,000 in England and Wales suffer from MS, but rates in Scotland are much higher at up to 190 per 100,000.

*Figure 10.1: My work was featured in The Sunday Times newspaper after helping a well known Scottish Actress Alison Peebles with Multiple Sclerosis (MS) get better and work again.*

That's how I met Gillian. Gillian had most of the symptoms with which people living with MS typically present. But she suffered particularly badly with her legs, where she experienced severe spasms. Often, her legs "wouldn't listen" to what she wanted them to do - and she would fall.

Gillian had been traveling to see me at my clinic for many months. My treatment had helped her and we had built a bond. But today, there was no treatment from me. Instead, Gillian was going to try BackHug, a robot I had designed and built that replicated my treatment. BackHug was a robotic clone of me and Gillian would be testing it.

The only analogy in literature for the suspense I felt that I can think of is… Frankenstein.

Using his scientific knowledge, Dr Frankenstein creates a copy of a living being. Using my engineering skills, I had created a robot that would give people like Gillian the treatment I had developed. Hopefully, my story would end better than Frankenstein's.

Now, to be fair, this wasn't the first robot I had developed. I had already produced a couple of versions with reasonably good results, including for people living with MS. But they were just prototypes. They delivered some benefits, but you couldn't say they fully replicated what I did with my hands.

\* \* \*

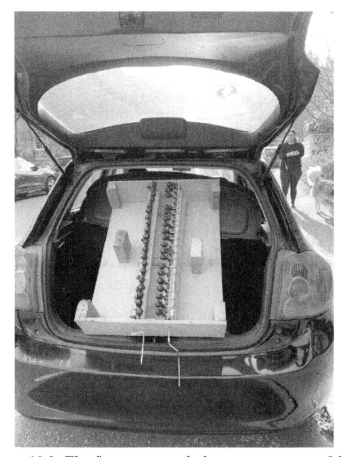

*Figure 10.2: The first ever proof-of-concept prototype I built in 2015. Since then, I kept it in my car boot for the last 7 years so it would remind me of how much progress I made from this rudimentary stage.*

There was a lot at stake. First, I had sunk all of the money I had made in the clinic into this project. Since 2015, I have spent all of my free time outside the clinic on this project. Then I had given up the steady income from my work as a physio to focus full time on this project. I was all in.

Now was my moment of truth.

(Well sort of).

Gillian is Scottish and, like other British people, the Scots are very polite. If a waitress asks them how their dinner was, they'll always say, "oh, it was great, thank you" - even if it was the worst meal they ever had and they can't wait to go home and give it one star on Tripadvisor. So when she said, "this is amazing," after her first BackHug session, I took it with a pinch of salt.

But then the text messages started coming. Her overall pain had reduced. The severe pain in her legs was almost gone. My head was spinning. When I called her the following week, she shared something that blew my mind. She had visited her MS nurse for a regular check-up. These appointments are designed, among other things, to monitor Gillian's progress against several benchmarks. Given Gillian's experience of falling, one of those benchmarks was how many falls she had had since the last appointment. When the nurse asked her that routine question Gillian stopped and realized she hadn't fallen!

This wasn't just British politeness! Gillian had been one of the patients whose condition had been most challenging for me to treat as a therapist, and she had been living with MS for almost three decades.

My manual treatment helped, but it was infrequent (Gillian lives a couple of hours drive from my old clinic.)

But now that she had a clone of me in her home that she could use every day, she was no longer suffering from the severe stiffness in her legs. The severe aches and pains that were debilitating her daily life had gone. She was actually walking in a much more stable way.

For years, I wondered whether I was completely crazy to have tried to create this robot clone of myself.

Then, a good friend of mine, Christopher Garner, 39 years senior to me, said to me, "It's your hands that do all the wonderful tricks. You have healing hands, and that fixes people's problems."

In one sense, I was flattered to hear the compliment. It made me feel a bit 'special' as a therapist. But, it didn't bode well for the device I would build.

Christopher tried a few early prototype versions and was not impressed "As I said, your hands do the job. I am skeptical that this machine can do what your hands could do."

It has been a constant battle between self-doubt and determination to prove the point that a machine can do the 'de-stiffening joints' job better than I do. So, when I witnessed how Gillian felt after using BackHug, all the doubts melted away. Gillian's experience alone made all of the money, sweat and stress worth it.

# WANT TO LIVE LIKE AN A-LISTER?

Imagine you were a Hollywood A-list actor or sold your startup to Apple or Google. You would have the money to hire me as your therapist. Everything you've learned so far in this book are secrets you can apply yourself, but it's also the secret of what you would get if you really became rich and famous and decided to spend some of your fortune on me as your live-in physio.

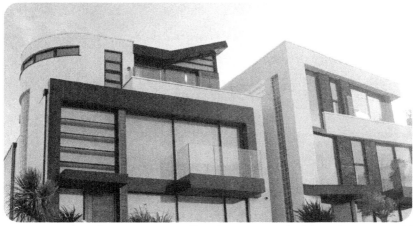

*Figure 10.3: If I were your live-in personal therapist, I would treat your neck and back to release joint stiffness, while dispensing advice on sitting straight and the right exercise to do. BackHug offers the same - or better - manual treatments than I ever could.*

\* \* \*

If I were your live-in personal therapist, we would have a conversation.

Then, I would investigate the stiffness in your neck, shoulder blades, back, and everything that could contribute to it. I'd then spend an hour or more every day, treating your neck and back to release your joint stiffness.

Of course, I would nag you with an action plan of everything you needed to do to prevent the worsening.

I would advise you to:
- Exercise
- Improve your posture
- Break your sitting cycle

The list would go on.

We would develop the regular exercise action plan together, you would agree to follow it and it would give you the results you were looking for.

That brings us to where we are now.

Most people are not A-list Hollywood celebrities or tech billionaires (but if you are, more power to you).

But, despite that, you now understand the principles behind the secrets in this book. And that understanding gives you power. You know that stiff joints in the neck and back have an impact that spreads through your whole body. And you know what to do to deal with that impact. You're empowered.

When I look back on my life, I have no regrets.

I went from a sick boy with a tube in his nose to a physio who could find the root cause of people's problems and developed a technique to fix them.

That's not bad.

But now I want to go further. We need to apply all the principles behind the secrets in this book to something real and build a comprehensive system that you can rely on.

# EPIPHANY MOMENT

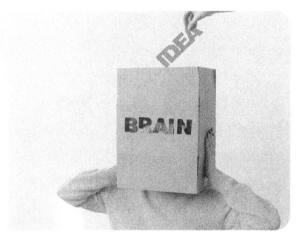

*Figure 10.4: I had a lightbulb moment thanks to a conversation with a friend in 2015, leading me to start developing BackHug.*

In this last section, I want to take you from being a passive recipient of knowledge to being a fully active and empowered participant, ready to experience the fully-functioning BackHug device on your own, in your own time and in a space of your choosing, and bring your chronic aches and pains to a definitive end.

Understanding the fundamental concepts and owning the treatment methods they result in is one of the most consequent things you can do for yourself.

Gillian understood the concepts and now holds the technique.

My goal in this last section is to offer you the tools

that you need to lead a healthier life and make that life even more enjoyable.

When I started this journey, I was still working at my day job as a physio. At the same time, I tried to build a machine that would do my work - releasing stiffness in the neck and back joints.

Why was I so desperate for this machine to work? As I described above, the only thing I had to deliver the signature technique which my patients were clamoring for was - my thumbs. It was those thumbs that applied the pressure to the stiff joints parts. And it was that pressure that released the stiffness. And the release of that joint stiffness gave my patients their lives back.

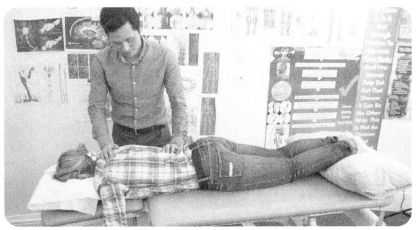

*Figure 10.5: I would see 6-10 patients a day, each spending 30 minutes working their back to release the joint stiffness in the*

*neck and back*

They would leave the clinic with a smile on their faces. But you can imagine how hard it was for me - doing that job every working day of the week (and Saturday), for eight hours, repeatedly. I couldn't do that for another five years, let alone a whole career. I really mean it, at some point, my thumbs would have fallen off.

Many of my patients had to travel long distances to visit my practice in Edinburgh. One of them traveled from Paris. Another one traveled from Egypt. Derek Smith lived in the outer Hebrides, on an island in the Atlantic ocean off the coast of Scotland. To get to my clinic, he had to fly for one hour on a small propeller plane and take a taxi from the airport to my practice.

He received his first session from me on the day he arrived. He then received the second session the day after, staying in a hotel overnight. After that, he had to go back home. Derek needed regular treatment. Flying to your therapist on a propeller plane was no way to do that.

One day he said to me, "Why don't you train someone on my island? Then I wouldn't have to travel." I thought, why not? I'm not someone who is motivated by money. Otherwise, I wouldn't have quit my well-paid job in engineering with Hyundai to become a physio. Plus I was overworked.

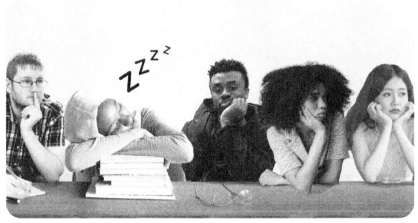

*Figure 10.6: I tried to train five other therapists with my own technique but they all found the technique too physically demanding, and it was too boring for them*

So I spent over the next six months trying to train five therapists, including one from Germany named Ben. To start, all of them thought it was a great idea.

They were full of enthusiasm.

But it didn't last.

My technique consists of repetitive movements.

Using those repetitive movements on spinal joints for nearly an hour, all day long, was physically very demanding.

And, to be honest, boring.

The trainees weren't enjoying it. If you asked them

how they saw their life over the next ten years, it didn't involve performing the same repetitive movement with their thumbs every working day of the year.

# HOW I CLONED MYSELF

One day, I went out for lunch with my late, dear friend, Kerry Napuk, to whom I have dedicated this book. Kerry was 39 years older than me, born the same year as my dad back in Korea. I have always enjoyed friendships with people who are much older than me. They are generous with their time, as well as great at sharing their wisdom and knowledge with younger friends.

On that day, I opened up. 'Kerry, my manual physiotherapy. It works. It works for my patients. It improves their lives. But it's hard. It's so hard. I thought I could train other people to do it for me, but no dice. It was just as hard for them. I don't want to do it. No one else wants to do it. But Kerry - someone needs to do it."

\* \* \*

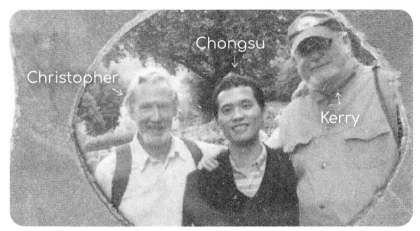

*Figure 10.7: Kerry, Christopher and me at "Dr Neil's Garden" in the village of Duddingston near Edinburgh, in 2014. Both Kerry and Christopher were 39 years older than me. We would go out for regular lunches and put the world to rights.*

Kerry had grown up watching Martin Luther King preaching and often talked about his experience of watching him deliver his famous speech near the Lincoln memorial in Washington DC in 1963 - known as the 'I have a dream' speech. He was passionate about everything from politics to food and healthcare and spoke with an eloquence that impressed me. When I told him about my difficulties he said, "The stuff you do, Chongsu, will always be hard to do. Unless you can get a machine to do it."

That was an EPIPHANY moment for me …

Why not?

After all, I trained as an engineer.

Why not make a machine that replicated what I was doing?

My patients could get all the benefits without my thumbs falling off.

A machine wouldn't get tired. As a result, the treatment would be consistent.

On top of that, the machine could have as many fingers as I wanted it to.

So, the machine would be the final piece of the jigsaw. It would enable widespread adoption of the theories supported by Kendall in his textbook and physiotherapy best practice in general, as championed by Maitland (summarised above in Secret #6). By taking the drudgery out of de-stiffening, it would remove the final barrier to widespread availability of the de-stiffening joints treatment that I and many other physiotherapists had discovered was the most effective way to help people with their pain.

I finally realized I could create a machine that could help so many people end their chronic aches and pains. No matter where they lived in the world or what their circumstances were, this machine could make them feel better by fixing the root of their problems.

The notion began to take a clear shape in my mind. It was a tall order, a huge challenge in fact, but I was determined to make it happen.

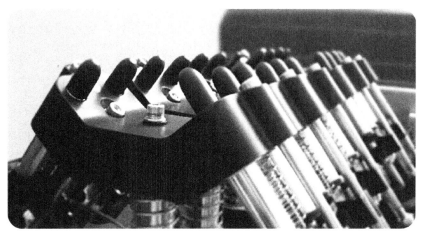

*Figure 10.8: The device could have as many fingers as I wanted it to, and it wouldn't get tired, giving consistent treatment all the time.*

And it could live in Derek's house, Gillian's house or the house of anyone who needed it. It would be there, on tap, for Derek or Gillian, or anyone else to use anytime, whenever they needed it. It seemed like a crazy project. Nothing like this had ever been attempted. There were so many questions to answer, so many risks. But nothing else was working. So I thought, why not?

That afternoon, I went straight down to the hardware store. I bought springs, bolts, nuts, and a piece of wood. Then, reactivating my engineering brain, I started working.

At the time, I was optimistic. I thought it would take me a couple of months. In fact, it took two years and a lot of money and energy before I finally produced my first working product. I was proud. I was sure it would impress the world.

But that's not how it worked out. Some people bought it, and it gave them some benefits (there are people with MS using it to this day). But it wasn't good enough. Not nearly. To be brutally honest, it was only 10-20% as good as what I believed it needed to be.

* * *

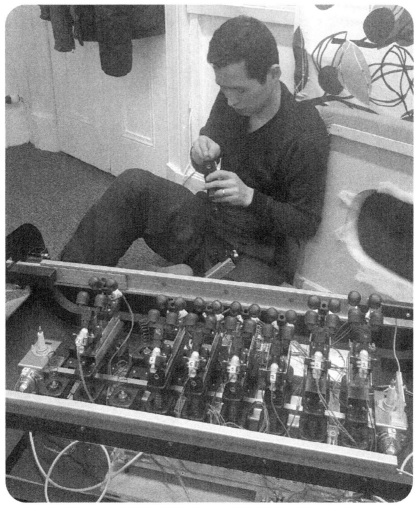

*Figure 10.9: Often I spent hours in the office till mid-night building and testing the early version of BackHug*

Looking back on my journey as an inventor, it's like peeling an onion. My first working product showed me how much I needed to improve the next version. The next showed me more things I needed to improve that I hadn't realized existed when I was building the first version, and so on, and so on.

When I thought of how much I needed to improve my invention and how hard that would be, I realized I wasn't going to be able to do it on my own. So over the next four years, I built a team around me: mechanical engineers, software engineers, graphic designers and more. We kept developing, testing, iterating. Building a team and setting up a project taught me a lot about being an entrepreneur (which was a whole new journey for me).

I will spare you the details, tweaks, frustrations, illuminations, adaptations that went into that journey. I think we must have made over 2,000 changes to the product I first developed, nearly running out of money a few times in the process. But, in 2022, seven years after the initial idea came up in 2015 over my lunch with Kerry, BackHug was born. Finally, we completed the development of a product that works and does what it's meant to do - more than I ever could with my thumbs.

It took seven years of relentless work, tinkering, crossing things out and starting all over again, to go from idea to sketches, from sketch to prototype and from prototype to finished product. But it was all worth it. Now, I can ethically market a life-changing product that has brought an end to chronic aches and pains for so many people around the world! That feels great.

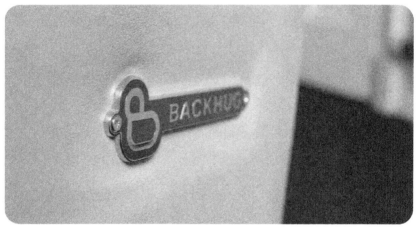

*Figure 10.10: In 2022, BackHug was launched after seven years of intensive research & development. The team and I took the initial idea through development to production.*

The next section is not meant to be a complete tutorial on using BackHug - you can find step-by-step instructions inside the BackHug App or in our video tutorials. Instead, I just want to focus on how simple it is to personalize BackHug to your individual requirements, empowering you to take control of your health, based on the fundamental principles in this book.

# CONNECT YOUR SMARTPHONE TO BACKHUG

The first step is to connect your smartphone to the BackHug device. Instead of having its own bespoke handset, we developed a dedicated App for BackHug so you can use your own smartphone as a handset, keeping things simple and giving you complete control over the treatment. The App offers you a neat and intuitive means of operating the device. Using a smartphone App rather than a specific piece of hardware means the App can get updated continuously, so you always get the most advanced control function.

* * *

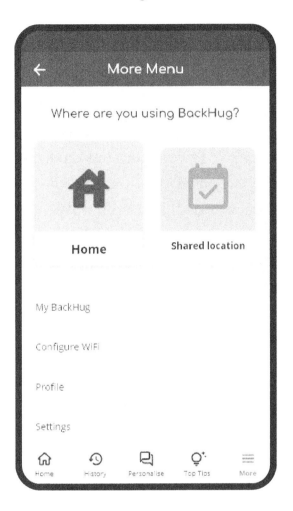

*Figure 10.11: BackHug is operated with a dedicated App which you download onto your smartphone. The App is simple to connect to your BackHug via Bluetooth, and you can use it on your smartphone as an easy-to-use handset to control the device*

Download the BackHug App on your smartphone from the Google or Apple Store and create your account. You will be asked about your height. This is so that the App can automatically select the number of treatment fingers to use depending on your back length, as part of an enhanced personalized treatment experience.

You then follow two simple steps to complete the connection between your smartphone and your BackHug

Add your BackHug device to your BackHug App.

Connect BackHug to your WiFi to enable the electronics on the device to be updated remotely and other features designed to optimize your treatment.

Once your BackHug is WiFi configured, it will stay connected to our cloud server. When there's new software available to improve personalization treatment features further, your machine will download the software immediately. Please note that, like with any piece of software, there will be cosmetic changes to BackHug App's user interface (UI) over time, so if the images you see when operating BackHug on your App don't look exactly the same as in this book, don't worry. The functionality will be the same - or better.

# TAKE THE IN-APP CHATBOT PHYSIO CONSULTATION

When you go and see a therapist, they will typically ask you a series of questions about the problem you came to see them about. Nutritionists will ask about your diet. Physiotherapists will ask about injuries or the part(s) of your body you feel pain in. And so on. Based on the information you provide, therapists will carefully determine what treatment program is best suited to solving your specific problem. For physiotherapists, those parameters would include the treatment type, area, intensity, duration and speed.

That is precisely what you will get from BackHug. On the App, all you need to do is start the in-App 1-1 software powered physiotherapy consultation. Just as in a consultation with a human therapist, you will be asked more than a dozen questions that are carefully designed to assess the treatment you need.

After you complete the questionnaire, the App processes the data using a specially designed algorithm based on the treatment methods I've been discussing in this book. The algorithm produces a unique treatment program just for you, to meet your individual needs.

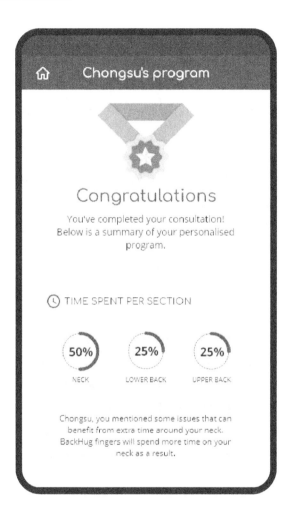

*Figure 10.12. On the BackHug App, when you complete the 1-1 chatbot physio consultation, you get a personalized treatment program that is specially made for you*

That personalized treatment program is stored on

your App so you can use the program next time you get on BackHug. I recommend you take a follow-up chatbot consultation at least every three months. Your back and the rest of your body will change and, in addition, the treatment will have a positive impact. By regularly updating your program, you will be making sure it's optimized for your current needs.

# THE FINGERS ADAPT TO YOUR BACK SHAPE

After creating a unique treatment program specifically tailored to your needs, you can get on the BackHug device and let the magic begin. We've made BackHug very intuitive so that non-techie people can use it. Most people get the hang of it right away, and it shouldn't take more than two sessions to become completely comfortable with the process. The very first thing that happens when you start the session, is the 'back scanning' feature:

You will feel the 26 robotic fingers underneath rise and gently touch your neck and back

Shortly after, the two fingers under the neck start moving. Follow the instructions on the App screen to adjust your body position, so you feel the two fingers touching the bottom of your skull.

Next, each pair of the robotic fingers starts scanning your entire back from the neck through the upper back to the lower back.

When the back scanning is complete, all 26 robotic fingers will be fixed.

\* \* \*

Each of the 26 fingers is now adapted to the individual shape of your back. Your back has a different shape from that of all of the other readers of this book. With the back scanning feature, BackHug's fingers will adopt a different configuration for your back and for the back of every other reader of this book.

\* \* \*

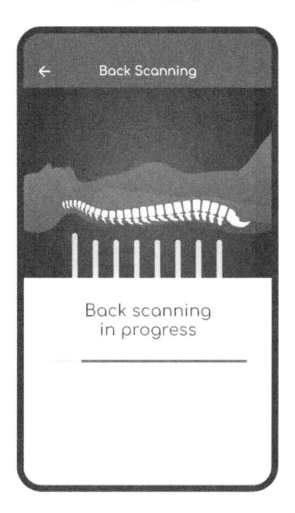

*Figure 10.13: Once you position yourself on the BackHug device, each of the 26 robotic fingers start scanning your back. The fingers adapt to the shape of your back so you get a personalized treatment experience*

# CUSTOMIZE YOUR TREATMENT ON THE APP

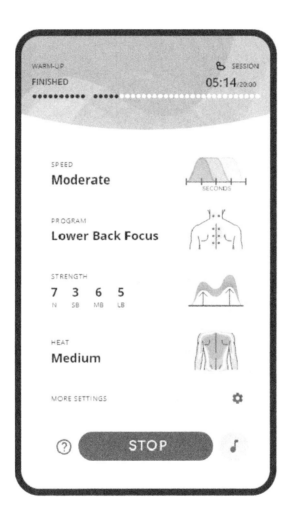

*Figure 10.14: The Settings on the BackHug App allows you to change speed, strength, area, duration and other functions in real-time.*

\* \* \*

One of my absolute favorite parts of BackHug is the Settings.

It's brilliant! It allows me to change how the BackHug is treating me instantly, in real-time. Although the in-App chatbot consultation produces a personalized treatment program for you, you can adjust the settings, such as the strength applied by the fingers to different parts of your back, to give you a treatment that's "just right" for how you're feeling in the moment.

On the BackHug App on your smartphone, it's very easy to understand how the Settings work and what to do. You use the App to choose the settings you prefer - it's that simple.

The Settings are: speed, strength, treatment area, back length and left-right balance.

Speed: The first step is to choose your treatment speed on the App screen: slow, medium or fast. Slow gives you a long stretch lasting more than 7 seconds with each finger stroke. Fast speed gives you a quick stretch lasting less than two seconds with each finger stroke.

\* \* \*

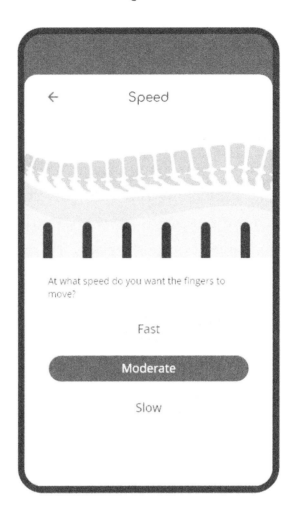

*Figure 10.15: You can choose one of three speeds to determine the stretching time. The slower the speed, the longer the stretch you experience.*

Strength: After you fix the speed, your next step is to select the strength of the pressure applied to each of the four parts of your back - neck, shoulder blades, upper back, and lower back. The strength setting determines how far the robotic fingers push. The higher you set the strength, the further and deeper the fingers push. For people with deep, tight knots, a good strong, deep push is just what you need. For people who have sensitive skin or lower tolerance thresholds, a strong push may be uncomfortable and softer pressure may feel better. We're all different. By offering the full range of strength settings - from 0 (off) to 10 (full power) - for each of the key parts of your back, BackHug is able to offer just the right level of strength to everyone. I would start on a low setting and gradually increase it to the point where it feels right. As a general rule, the stronger the pressure you can take, the more benefits you get. But you should never feel uncomfortable. Remember, you can adjust the strength in real time so, if you ever feel uncomfortable, just reduce it, and if your back is looser and you can take a stronger push, just increase it.

* * *

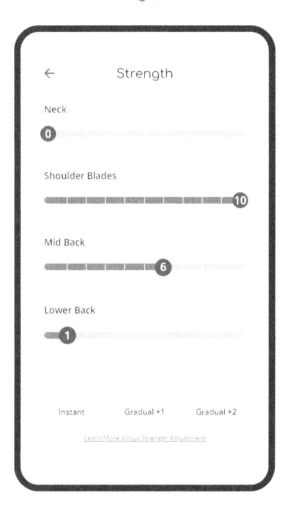

*Figure 10.16: The 'strength' setting has 10 different levels to choose from. You can select different strength settings for each of the four treatment areas. Selecting 0 means you'll get no treatment at all at that particular part of your back while choosing 10 means you get the strongest pressure possible.*

Treatment area: There are four different treatment sections you can choose - neck, shoulder blades, upper back, and lower back. But you only get treatment there if you choose to. You can activate or deactivate treatment in any area with the strength selector. To activate treatment in any of these four parts, for example your lower back, simply make sure the 'strength' setting is at 1 or above. But if you don't want any treatment at all in one of those areas, for example your neck, all you have to do is slide the 'strength' setting for that particular part of your body to zero ('0').

* * *

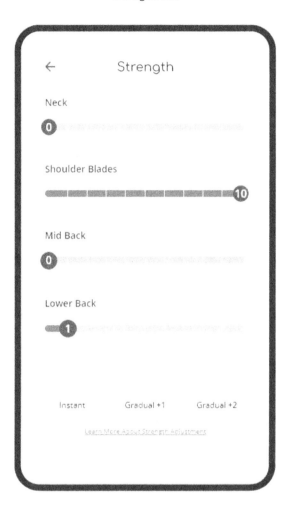

*Figure 10.17: If you don't want any treatment at all in a particular area, slide the 'strength' to zero '0' on the slide for that particular area*

Back length: One of the neatest things about the Setting Adjustor is that you can select how far down your lower back the treatment goes. When you create a BackHug account, you will be asked what your height is (don't worry, it doesn't have to be accurate to the inch). Depending on the height you input, the machine adjusts the number of treatment fingers which will work on your back.

As a rule of thumb, if you are 5ft 11" (180 centimeters) or taller, then your back is "long" enough to be treated by all the fingers and the pair of fingers at the very bottom will remain switched on. But if you're less than 5ft 11" tall, the two fingers at the bottom will be switched off. The reason for that is, simply, that the bottom two fingers will tend to be uncomfortable for you if you are less than 5ft 11" and they wouldn't give you much therapeutic benefit. Please note this is only a rough rule of thumb because back length can vary a lot independently from overall height. You can think of overall height as the combination of the length of your legs, your back and your head. Some people can have long legs and a short back, and vice versa. If you're not sure, try with the lower fingers on and off and see which you like best. If the lower fingers are uncomfortable you can switch them off anytime.

* * *

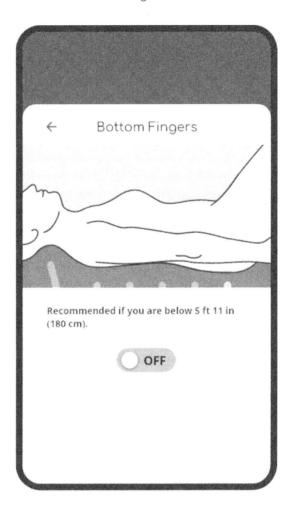

*Figure 10.18: You can switch the last pair of treatment fingers on or off depending on your back length*

Left & right balance: After choosing all the other settings, you can, if you wish, adjust the 'left & right balance' setting. Most people tend to want as much treatment on their left as on their right. But quite a lot of people are particularly sensitive on one side, or need extra treatment on the other. For example, if you're left handed you usually have more tension on the left side of your back, while right handed people have more on the right side. If your back is curved to either side, if you suffer from scoliosis like Soo does for example (see Secret #4), one side of your back will have more tension than the other. In cases like these, BackHug lets you choose to have stronger treatment on the side with the most tension.

* * *

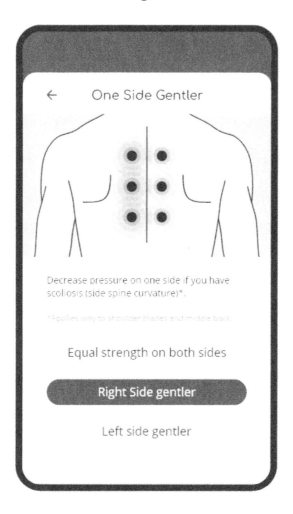

*Figure 10.19: If one side of your back is more tense, you can choose to have stronger treatment on that side*

The settings are simple and intuitive to adjust, but there are solid therapeutic reasons for consciously adjusting them so that you get a personalized treatment that really works for you.

# BACK TENSION TRACKING TO MONITOR YOUR PROGRESS

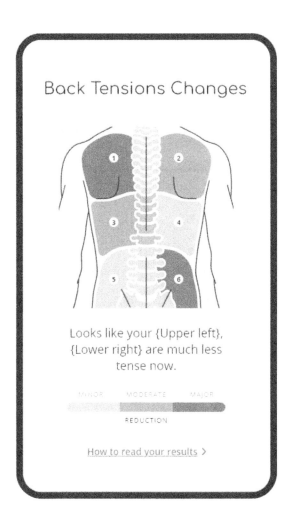

*Figure 10.20: Back Tension Tracking analyses how much back tension has changed during the session in real-time. Each of the six zones are analysed and processed in our server algorithm*

---

\* \* \*

As excellent as the BackHug device and App are at offering you personalized treatment at your fingertips, it only matters if you experience a reduction in your back stiffness during the session and over time as you keep using BackHug.

Sure, BackHug can create a uniquely tailored treatment program for me with the in-App consultation, and I can adjust the settings to adapt treatment to what I need on any given day. But what ultimately gives you satisfaction as a user, what "gives you your life back" (pun intended), is the increase in your back relaxation and reduction in back tension you achieve with each BackHug session.

That's why I created Back Tension Tracking, a groundbreaking software feature that has been developed for over two years. You can use Back Tension Tracking to track how much your back has relaxed during BackHug treatment and, crucially, monitor your progress over time. So far as I am aware, this is the first time software has been able to measure back tension or relaxation on an industrial scale. As we have seen throughout this book, back relaxation happens as a result of de-stiffening the joints in the back, and de-stiffening helps with aches and pains in the neck, back, head, arms and legs. It also improves

264

energy levels, flexibility and leg stiffness and helps you breathe deeply, which enables you to relax or meditate.

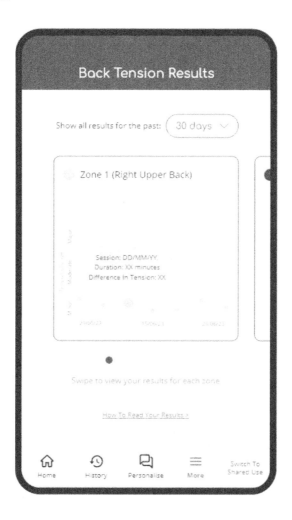

*Figure 10.21: This is an example that the user would see at the end of their session. It shows how much back tension has changed during their session. For the algorithm to be able to analyse sufficient amount of data, the treatment duration has to*

*be minimum 20 minutes long*

In 2021, we carried out a scientific study to evaluate how effective BackHug is for releasing stiff back muscles. We used Myoton Pro, a device scientifically proven to measure changes in muscle stiffness. The results were impressive. They showed that, on average, each BackHug session reduced back muscle stiffness 3.7X times MORE than what was experienced by the control group who were simply resting in bed. Not just that. Participants reported an average 44% reduction in their subjective level of aches, pains, and discomfort after three BackHug sessions.

We knew we had a truly revolutionary product, but those results even shocked me. We knew we designed a product that "seemed" to work on pretty much every person that used it. But now, through the use of a Myoton Pro device, it showed the product really reduced stiffness - there is objective proof that BackHug works.

* * *

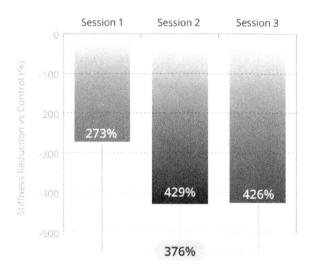

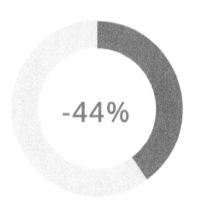

*Figure 10.22: It was important to test whether BackHug works scientifically, so we conducted a study using the Myoton Pro device. The study showed 371% greater stiffness reduction in the BackHug group*

Myoton is a very expensive device and you can't

use it on yourself. Even if someone else is using it on you it's hard to do without a physiotherapy table to lie down on. But with Back Tension Tracking, you are empowered to measure your own progress and track what BackHug is doing for you, purely via a software solution. Who knows, maybe in the future we will be able to use the data from Back Tension Tracking to further optimize and personalize BackHug treatment for each individual BackHug user, perhaps using AI. That futuristic chapter of our story has yet to be written but stay tuned.

# USE WHENEVER YOU NEED

After you've tried a few treatment sessions on BackHug, you'll notice that each hardware feature and software is optimized to create the most effective personalized treatment experience.

As you become familiar with the type of treatment you're getting from BackHug, you can start experimenting with different settings to increase the benefits further.

However, even if you feel great after a few months of BackHug use, it's a good idea to keep using it from time to time to stay loose and flexible so you avoid the tension building up again. Remember, unless your body is looked after regularly, the joints will become rusty, which will then cause the development of many problems as you age.

You will get therapeutic results in record time! Isn't that amazing?! While this would have taken my one-to-one physiotherapy two to three months to achieve the same level, you can now experience the benefits from BackHug in about a few sessions.

If you don't have your BackHug device yet, you can get a 30-day risk-free trial at www.mybackhug.com so you can get started right away.

# CONCLUSION

I ran a physiotherapy clinic for almost seven years before I decided that I needed to stop completely. I chose to put my vocation on pause so I could focus my energy on developing BackHug and making sure my robotic clone would be a success. Seven years on from that decision, my team of engineers and I completed the development of the device, and started shipping it to many impatient customers across the UK, who had all been waiting a long time for something to ease their aches and pains in a sustainable way.

Having made thousands of changes to the initial version of the product, I was nervous about whether it would be up to the job, and whether it would really work for people suffering aches and pains.

Given the stage of our development, we could only release a limited number of BackHug devices, which meant we couldn't supply everyone who wanted one. That was frustrating. We felt that the best solution was to interview prospective customers on the phone or by email to get a comprehensive understanding of their needs and what their situation was, so devices could be shipped to those who would get the most benefit from using BackHug.

One of our prospective customers was a very young man. I wasn't sure he would be the right fit, since most people only develop a bad back after reaching a certain age.

Sean completely changed the way I understand back pain, even after over a decade in the field. He graduated from college only a year ago and started working as an analyst in a finance company. He explained that he had been quietly suffering a lot from severe aches and pains since his college years. His symptoms were so severe that he had to spend at least one hour stretching to ease the tension every day. The tightness he was experiencing in his back meant he could only breathe at chest level and couldn't achieve deep abdominal breathing. Only if he was able to visit the chiropractor for an adjustment a few times a week would he be able to achieve deep abdominal breathing.

"I managed to keep it at bay during the college years because I had the time and the flexibility to take time off and do stretching almost every day. And I didn't need to sit down for too long. But, when I started working, the problem hit me big time. I was spending eight hours sitting in the office, which completely seized up my back. Towards the end of the day, the pain would be so severe that I was thinking about looking for a different line of work," he says.

"I had no life after work. I couldn't go out for a drink. I couldn't meet with my friends because I was spending all my free time keeping the pain at bay. I'd be going to a physiotherapist or chiropractor three times every week to get my back sorted. That's a lot of money and loads of time I could have been doing other things, having a life basically. After treatment, I felt better and could breathe more deeply. But if I couldn't go for treatment, I would spend at least an hour stretching my back and legs in the evening. That's all I had. No fun!"

"I remember six months ago, I was on a call with someone who worked at BackHug. When he said this thing fixed bad backs I was obviously keen to find out more. Because I'd suffered for so long, I'd almost become an expert on back problems. I tried everything: massage gun, massage chair, handheld massager, acupuncture, chiropractor, physio, you name it. Because of that experience I was skeptical. 'But does this thing really work?' I asked. The guy was adamant, he was a user himself, as well as an employee. He'd seen the impact on other customers. He didn't have any doubt. At the same time, he was working for the company, so he was hardly impartial.

But they offered a 30-day trial after which you could return it if it didn't work. That was good enough for me and I gave it a try. And I'm so glad I did. It gave my life back. I mean, literally, I now have a life outside of work and back care. It's great."

I was very moved by what he said. I never expected someone so young to know what it's like to live in constant pain. As with so many of my patients, nothing showed up in any medical examination. The doctors just couldn't help him.

If you haven't tried BackHug yet, you'll discover its benefits very fast as soon as you start using it. Like Sean, you may feel there's no hope. You may feel condemned to living the rest of your life oppressed by constant aches and pains. But now you know there's a solution. It's available to you 24/7, in the convenience of your own home, saving you a bundle of money and time.

I'm so grateful that you've taken the plunge, that you've invested the time and patience to follow me on this journey. You have taken an active decision to take control of your health and that's great. Nothing is more important than your health and wellbeing. If you look after your body well, and if you have a solution you can trust 100%, then you have set yourself free from the aches and pains that have been holding you back for so long.

Remember, this is a guidebook. Don't just read it once and then go back to business as usual. It's incredible how quickly you go back to square one if you relapse into bad habits. Keep it handy, and reread to refresh your understanding. This book is a reminder and a guide for your health and that of your beloved family.

I hope that you can use these secrets to understand more about your own body and look after it. By now you will have realized how much that's in your best interest. Your body is constantly giving you signals - telling you when there are problems. Once it does that, it's going to be waiting for you to do something about it. To do something to make your body healthy again. If you follow and stay true to that basic principle, your life will be full of energy and hope, and you really will live your life to the fullest.

Thank you for allowing me to serve you through this book. It's truly been a great honor, and I am really looking forward to seeing how you do with the 'de-stiffening joints' frameworks you've learned. Come visit me on any of my social media platforms, say hello, and please share with me how these 'secrets' have changed your life.

* * *

Thanks,
Chongsu Lee

P.S. Don't forget, you're just one solution away…

# WORKS CITED

i.   Adstrum, Sue, et al. "Defining the fascial system." Journal of Bodywork and Movement Therapies, vol. 21, no. 1, 2017, pp. 173-177. Science Direct, https://www.sciencedirect.com/science/article/abs/pii/S1360859216302595.

ii.  Ballestero-Pérez, Ruth, et al. "Effectiveness of Nerve Gliding Exercises on Carpal Tunnel Syndrome: A Systematic Review." J Manipulative Physiol Ther ., vol. 40, no. 1, 2017, pp. 50-59. Pubmed NCBI, https://pubmed.ncbi.nlm.nih.gov/27842937/.

iii. Brennan, Dan. "Fascia: Layers, Pain, and Treatment." WebMD, 20 June 2021, https://www.webmd.com/a-to-z-guides/what-is-fascia. Accessed 4 May 2022.

iv.  Chang, Wen-Dien, et al. "Core strength training for patients with chronic low back pain." J Phys Ther Sci, vol. 27, no. 3, 2015, pp. 619–622. US National Library of Medicine National Institutes of Health, https://www.ncbi.nlm.nih.gov/pmc/articles/PMC4395677/.

v.   Chiarello, Cynthia. Physical Rehabilitation Evidence-Based Examination, Evaluation, and

Intervention. ELSEVIER, 2007. ScienceDirect, https://www.sciencedirect.com/science/article/pii/B9780721603612500119.

vi. Dalley, Arthur F., et al. Clinically Oriented Anatomy. Lippincott Williams & Wilkins, 2006.

vii. Ebraheim. M.D., Nabil. "Body Positions Affecting the spine and discs - Everything You Need To Know - Nabil Ebraheim, M.D." YouTube, 20 August 2010, https://youtu.be/_T-eQJnZRRk. Accessed 13 March 2022.

viii. Eidelson, Stewart G., et al. "Upper Back Pain Center - Symptoms Causes Treatments." SpineUniverse, 4 May 2021, https://www.spineuniverse.com/conditions/upper-back-pain. Accessed 2 March 2022.

ix. Hansraj, KK. "Assessment of stresses in the cervical spine caused by posture and position of the head." Surg Technol Int, vol. Nov, no. 25, 2014, pp. 277-9. National Library of Medicine, https://pubmed.ncbi.nlm.nih.gov/25393825/.

x. Hasebe, Kiyotaka, et al. "The effect of dynamic stretching on hamstrings flexibility with respect to the spino-pelvic rhythm." The Journal of Medical Investigation, vol. 63, no. 1.2, 2016, pp. 85-90. J-STAGE, https://www.jstage.jst.go.jp/article/jmi/63/1.2/63_85/_article.

xi. https://health.gov/sites/default/files/
2 0 1 9 - 0 9 /
Physical_Activity_Guidelines_2nd_edition.pdf.
"Physical Activity Guidelines for Americans,
2nd edition." Office of Disease Prevention and
Health Promotion, 2018, https://health.gov/
s i t e s / d e f a u l t / f i l e s / 2 0 1 9 - 0 9 /
Physical_Activity_Guidelines_2nd_edition.pdf.
Accessed 13 May 2022.

xii. Hvedstrup, Jeppe, et al. "Increased neck muscle
stiffness in migraine patients with ictal neck
pain: A shear wave elastography study."
Cephalalgia: International journal of headache,
vol. 40, no. (6), 2020, pp. 565-574. pubmed.gov,
https://pubmed.ncbi.nlm.nih.gov/32295400/
#affiliation-1.

xiii. Kendall, Florence Peterson, et al. Muscles:
Testing and Function with Posture and Pain.
Edited by Florence Peterson Kendall, Lippincott
Williams & Wilkins, 2005.

xiv. Kingston, Laura, et al. "The effects of spinal
mobilizations on the sympathetic nervous
system: a systematic review." Manual Therapy,
vol. 19, no. 4, 2014, pp. 281-7. NIH National
L i b r a r y  o f  M e d i c i n e ,  h t t p s : / /
pubmed.ncbi.nlm.nih.gov/24814903/.

xv. L.Brininger, MAJ Teresa, et al. "Efficacy of a Fabricated Customized Splint and Tendon and Nerve Gliding Exercises for the Treatment of Carpal Tunnel Syndrome: A Randomized Controlled Trial." Archives of Physical Medicine and Rehabilitation, vol. 88, no. 11, 2007, pp. 1429-1435. Science Direct, https://www.sciencedirect.com/science/article/abs/pii/S0003999307013378.

xvi. Lee, Keun-Su, and Joon-Hee Lee. "Effect of maitland mobilization in cervical and thoracic spine and therapeutic exercise on functional impairment in individuals with chronic neck pain." J Phys Ther Sci., vol. 29, no. 3, 2017, pp. 531–535. National Library of Medicine, https://www.ncbi.nlm.nih.gov/pmc/articles/PMC5361027/.

xvii. Levine, James A. Get Up! Why Your Chair is Killing You and What You Can Do About It. St. Martin's Publishing Group, 2014.

xviii. Li, Jun, et al. "Musculoskeletal Pain in Parkinson's Disease." Frontiers in Neurology, vol. 12, no. 1, 2022, pp. 1-8. Frontiers, https://www.frontiersin.org/articles/10.3389/fneur.2021.756538/full.

xix. LOR physical therapy. "Tight Chest Muscles:

Why Your Upper Back Is the Key to Their Release — Laguna Orthopedic Rehabilitation." Laguna Orthopedic Rehabilitation, 24 July 2019, https://www.lorpt.com/blog/2019/7/24/chest-muscle-tightness-back-related. Accessed 12 March 2022.

xx. Louw, Maryke. "Understanding how your nerves may affect/cause Achilles tendinopathy." TREAT MY ACHILLES, 2019, https://www.treatmyachilles.com/post/understanding-how-your-nerves-may-affect-cause-achilles-tendinopathy. Accessed 06 03 2022.

xxi. Luca, A., Nicoletti, A., Mostile, G., & Zappia, M. (2019). The Parkinsonian Personality: More Than Just a "Trait". Frontiers in neurology, 9, 1191. https://doi.org/10.3389/fneur.2018.01191. Accessed 17 August 2023

xxii. Maitland, Geoffrey Douglas. Vertebral Manipulation. Butterworths, 1977.

xxiii. Mandell, Alan. "Dr Mandell's Atlanto-Occipital Fix for Headaches, Neck Pain, Trap, Interscapular, Dizziness, Visual." YouTube, 21 November 2016, https://youtu.be/Z82rkyj8n_c. Accessed 12 March 2022.

xxiv. Mistry, Gopi, and Neeta Vyas.

"Comparison of hamstrings flexibility in subjects with chronic low back pain versus normal individuals." Journal of Clinical &amp Experimental Research, vol. 2, no. (1), 2014, p. 85. ResearchGate, https://www.researchgate.net/publication/272666204_Comparison_of_hamstrings_flexibility_in_subjects_with_chronic_low_back_pain_versus_normal_individuals.

xxv. NICE Guideline. "Recommendations | Parkinson's disease in adults | Guidance." NICE, 19 July 2017, https://www.nice.org.uk/guidance/ng71/chapter/Recommendations#non-pharmacological-management-of-motor-and-non-motor-symptoms. Accessed 21 November 2022.

xxvi.     Nimwegen, Marlies van, et al. "Physical inactivity in Parkinson's disease." Journal of Neurology, vol. 258, no. 12, 2011, 2214–2221. National Library of Medicine, https://www.ncbi.nlm.nih.gov/pmc/articles/PMC3225631/.

xxvii.     Ocran, Edwin. "Joints and ligaments of the vertebral column." Kenhub, https://www.kenhub.com/en/library/anatomy/joints-and-ligaments-of-the-vertebral-column.

Accessed 10 November 2022.

xxviii.    Ogoke, B. "The management of the atlanto-occipital and atlanto-axial joint pain." Pain Physician, vol. 3, no. 3, 2000, pp. 289–293. PubMed, https://pubmed.ncbi.nlm.nih.gov/16906186/.

xxix.    Ogoke, Bentley A. "The Management of the Atlanto-Occipital and Atlanto-Axial Joint Pain." Pain Physician ., vol. 3, no. 3, 2000, pp. 289-293. PubMed.gov, https://www.painphysicianjournal.com/linkout?issn=1533-3159&vol=3&page=289.

xxx.Ohrnberger, Julius, et al. "The relationship between physical and mental health: A mediation analysis." Social Science & Medicine, vol. 195, no. 1, 2017, pp. 42-49.

xxxi.    Parkinson's UK. "What is Parkinson's?" Parkinson's UK, 2022, https://www.parkinsons.org.uk/information-and-support/what-parkinsons. Accessed 21 November 2022.

xxxii.    Reis, Felipe Jose Jandre, and Adriana Ribeiro Macedo. "Influence of Hamstring Tightness in Pelvic, Lumbar and Trunk Range of Motion in Low Back Pain and Asymptomatic Volunteers during Forward Bending." Asian

Spine J, vol. (4), no. (4), 2015, 535–540. NCBI, https://www.ncbi.nlm.nih.gov/pmc/articles/PMC4522442/.

xxxiii.    Rutten, Geert M., et al. "Interrupting long periods of sitting: good STUFF." Int J Behav Nutr Phys Act., vol. 10, no. 1, 2013, pp. 1-10. US National Library of Medicine National Institutes of Health, https://www.ncbi.nlm.nih.gov/pmc/articles/PMC3542098/.

xxxiv.    Shah, Shlesha G., and Vijay Kage. "Effect of Seven Sessions of Posterior-to-Anterior Spinal Mobilisation versus Prone Press-ups in Non-Specific Low Back Pain – Randomized Clinical Trial." J Clin Diagn Res, vol. 10, no. 3, 2016, YC10–YC13. National Library of Medicine, https://www.ncbi.nlm.nih.gov/pmc/articles/PMC4843372/.

xxxv.    Shakya, Nishchal Ratna, and Sajan Manandhar. "Prevalence of hamstring muscle tightness among undergraduate physiotherapy students of Nepal using passive knee extension angle test." International Journal of Scientific and Research Publications, vol. 8, no. 1, 2018, pp. 182–185. IJSPR.ORG, http://www.ijsrp.org/research-paper-0118.php?rp=P737129.

xxxvi.    Soames, Roger, et al. Anatomy and

Human Movement: Structure and Function. Butterworth Heinmann/Elsevier, 2006.

xxxvii.     Tak, Sajin, et al. "The effects of active release technique on the gluteus medius for pain relief in persons with chronic low back pain." Phys Ther Rehabil Sci, vol. 2, no. (1), 2013, pp. 27-30. PHYSICAL THERAPY REHABILITATION SCIENCE, https://doi.org/10.14474/ptrs.2013.2.1.27.

xxxviii.    Trijffel, Emiel van, et al. "Are Changes in Synovial Fluid Volume or Distribution a Determinant of Biomechanical Effects of Passive Joint Movements?" International Musculoskeletal Medicine, vol. 38, no. 3-4, 2016, pp. 115-121. ResearchGate, https://www.researchgate.net/publication/312020838_Are_Changes_in_Synovial_Fluid_Volume_or_Distribution_a_Determinant_of_Biomechanical_Effects_of_Passive_Joint_Movements_-_International_Musculoskeletal_Medicine_2016 383-4115-121.

xxxix.      Volpi, Elena, et al. "Muscle tissue changes with aging." Curr Opin Clin Nutr Metab Care., vol. 7, no. 4, 2004, pp. 405–410. NIH Public Access, https://www.ncbi.nlm.nih.gov/pmc/articles/PMC2804956/pdf/nihms131937.pdf.

xl. Walsh, Mart T. "Upper Limb Neural Tension Testing and Mobilization: Fact, Fiction, and a Practical Approach." Journal of Hand Therapy, vol. 18, no. 2, 2005, pp. 241-258. Science Direct, https://www.sciencedirect.com/science/article/abs/pii/S0894113005000505.

xli. Webborn, Nick. "A Neuropathic Model to the Etiology and Management of Achilles Tendinopathy." Wiley Online Library, Wiley, 2007, https://onlinelibrary.wiley.com/doi/10.1002/9780470757987.ch10. Accessed 06 03 2022.

xlii. WHO. "Musculoskeletal conditions." WHO | World Health Organization, 8 February 2021, https://www.who.int/news-room/fact-sheets/detail/musculoskeletal-conditions. Accessed 16 April 2022.

xliii. Zeigelboim, Bianca, et al. "Neurotological Findings at a Health Unit for Adults with Cervicalgia." Int Arch Otorhinolaryngol., vol. 20, no. (2), 2016, pp. 109-113. NCBI resources, https://www.ncbi.nlm.nih.gov/pmc/articles/PMC4835335/.

# ABOUT THE AUTHOR

Chongsu Lee started developing Backhug while he was running a physiotherapy clinic in Edinburgh. During his first two years of practice, he discovered a unique hands-on treatment method which alleviated people's chronic aches and pains very successfully. People began to notice, and he was soon attracting patients from across the U.K and even as far as France and Egypt. Over the last 12 years, he has tried, tested and refined his manual technique, helped his patients get their life back on track, popularized the concept of de-stiffening joints, and founded the robotic company BackHug, which has helped thousands of aches and pains sufferers get better quickly. He lives in Edinburgh with his family, and you can reach out to him online at facebook.com/chongsu.lee.7.

Printed in Great Britain
by Amazon

26868622R00165